Narratives of recovery from mental illness

Narratives of recovery from mental illness presents research that challenges the prevailing view that recovery from 'mental illness' must take place within the boundaries of traditional mental health services. While Watts and Higgins accept that medical treatment may be a start to some people's recovery, they argue that mental health problems can also be resolved through everyday social interactions and through peer and community support.

Using a narrative approach, this book presents detailed recovery stories of 26 people who received various diagnoses of 'mental illness' and were involved in a mutual-help group known as GROW. Drawing on an in-depth analysis of each story, chapters offer new understandings of the journey into mental distress and a progressive entrapment through a combination of events, feelings, thoughts and relationships. The book also discusses the process of ongoing personal liberation and healing which assists recovery and suggests that friendship, social involvement, compassion and nurturing processes of change are all key factors in improved mental well-being.

This book provides an alternative way of looking at 'mental illness' and demonstrates many unexplored avenues and paths to recovery that need to be considered. As such, it will be of interest to researchers, academics and postgraduate students in the fields of psychiatry, psychology, nursing, social work and occupational therapy, as well as to service providers, policy makers and peer-support organisations. The narratives of recovery within the book should also be a source of hope to people struggling with 'mental illness' and emotional distress.

Mike Watts was, for many years, the National Program Coordinator for GROW in Ireland. Based in Kilkenny, he is currently involved in recovery research and works with diverse groups of service users, family members, mental health professionals, students and policy makers as part of a national endeavour to create a recovery-oriented mental health service.

Agnes Higgins has worked in the area of mental health practice and education for more than 30 years and is currently Professor in Mental Health at the School of Nursing and Midwifery, Trinity College Dublin, Ireland. She is involved in a number of research projects that are advancing understanding of the recovery experiences of people who experience mental health problems, as well as providing templates of collaborative and empowering research methods.

Advances in mental health research series

Books in this series:

The clinical effectiveness of neurolinguistic programming
A Critical Appraisal
Edited by Lisa Wake, Richard M. Gray & Frank S. Bourke

Group therapy for adults with severe mental illness
Adapting the Tavistock method
Diana Semmelhack, Larry Ende & Clive Hazell

Narratives of art practice and mental wellbeing
Reparation and connection
Olivia Sagan

Video and filmmaking as psychotherapy
Research and practice
Edited by Joshua L. Cohen and J. Lauren Johnson with Penelope P. Orr

Schizotypy
New dimensions
Edited by Oliver Mason and Gordon Claridge

The prevention of suicide in prison
Cognitive behavioural approaches
Edited by Daniel Pratt

Narratives of recovery from mental illness
The role of peer support
Mike Watts and Agnes Higgins

Narratives of recovery from mental illness

The role of peer support

Mike Watts and Agnes Higgins

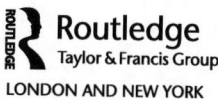

Routledge
Taylor & Francis Group

LONDON AND NEW YORK

First published 2017
by Routledge
2 Park Square, Milton Park, Abingdon, Oxon OX14 4RN

and by Routledge
605 Third Avenue, New York, NY 10017

First issued in paperback 2022

Routledge is an imprint of the Taylor & Francis Group, an informa business

Publisher's Note
The publisher has gone to great lengths to ensure the quality of this reprint but points out that some imperfections in the original copies may be apparent.

British Library Cataloguing in Publication Data
A catalogue record for this book is available from the British Library

Library of Congress Cataloging-in-Publication Data
Names: Watts, Mike, Ph. D., author. | Higgins, Agnes, author.
Title: Narratives of recovery from mental illness : the role of peer support / Mike Watts and Agnes Higgins.
Description: Abingdon, Oxon ; New York, NY : Routledge, 2017. | Includes bibliographical references.
Identifiers: LCCN 2016007302 | ISBN 9781138847996 (hardcover) | ISBN 9781315726243 (electronic)
Subjects: | MESH: Mental Disorders—rehabilitation | Mental Disorders—psychology | Self-Help Groups | Peer Group | Social Support | Personal Narratives
Classification: LCC RC480.5 | NLM WM 400 | DDC 616.89/1—dc23
LC record available at http://lccn.loc.gov/2016007302

ISBN: 978-1-03-240244-4 (pbk)
ISBN: 978-1-138-84799-6 (hbk)
ISBN: 978-1-315-72624-3 (ebk)

DOI: 10.4324/9781315726243

Typeset in Times New Roman
by Apex CoVantage, LLC

Contents

SECTION 3

Figures

Foreword

Carol Mussey

In their book on recovery and peer support, Mike Watts and Agnes Higgins, along with their 26 recovered collaborators, argue persuasively that recovery from extreme distress or 'mental illness' is a real and ordinary human process, not a mystery to be deciphered only by 'brain disease' experts. This book should be read by anyone who is searching for a hopeful, person-centred approach to the healing of human distress.

How better to learn about the true path of recovery than from the lived experiences of those who have struggled down isolated roads of terror and gradually found their way back to a 're-enchantment with life'? By sitting with and carefully studying the stories of 26 recovered members of the peer-support organisation known as GROW, Mike and Agnes were able to map the complex way of recovery and personal growth. The journey begins with friendly acceptance and careful listening by others; progresses to relationships that are mutually supportive and challenging; develops further into self-activation, empowerment, reasonable risk taking and leadership; and finally extends to meaningful social involvement beyond the peer-support community.

The authors argue for a mental health system in which the professional is not 'on top but on tap' (GROW 2001:52) and the recovering person is progressively activated to become the agent for his or her own healing. Mike and Agnes are not so much arguing against professional mental health care (including medical intervention) as they are advocating for a more comprehensive and respectful view of the person in distress. Struggling individuals are not the mere product of a faulty brain. Rather, they have become the persons they are today through complex causes that demand complex solutions.

This book helps de-mystify the recovery process, revealing a human journey that is not unique to those who have been diagnosed with a 'mental illness'. Who among us has not struggled to recover from some form of distress – like the loss of a loved one, a debilitating illness or accident, abandonment, betrayal, war, trauma, violence, abuse or addiction? During dark times, haven't we too needed someone to listen with compassion to our story, inspire hopefulness and remind us of our resilience?

As the authors assert, peer-support programs with their alternative message need to be included as equal partners in an effective mental health system.

'Service users' often hear the message, 'You need our help and always will'. The peer-support message rings differently – 'We are here to help you, and eventually you will also learn to help others'. Organizations like GROW need the active involvement of their members in order to be effective, which means they need their members as much as their members need them. It is these reciprocal relationships that best support the healing process.

This book, with its poetic undertones, is recommended to anyone who is searching for a deeper, more compassionate understanding of the causes and solutions to human distress. All of us have something to learn when it comes to our common human challenges.

I am especially enthusiastic about endorsing this book since I achieved my own recovery from 'mental illness' through GROW. Still today I continue to benefit from new GROW opportunities that allow me to keep growing into 'freedom and wholeness' (GROW 2001:24).

Carol Mussey
International Program Coordinator
GROW International
USA 2016

Foreword

Jacqui Dillon

The therapeutic concept of recovery within mental health has been crucial in providing a much-needed antidote to the simplistic and pessimistic premise that human misery and distress are caused by chemical imbalances and genetic predispositions, as propagated by biomedical psychiatry and the pharmaceutical industries. The knowledge that people *can and do* recover from serious mental health issues has provided a much-needed sense of optimism about the possibility of change, healing and growth.

However, there is a danger that as recovery becomes more widely adopted within mainstream mental health services, the concept is being colonised, so that its most radical aspects are assimilated, and it simply becomes another method of controlling and coercing people under the guise of offering something innovative and empowering. As well as this, the concept of recovery can individualise social problems, diverting attention from addressing urgent social and economic problems, which frequently underlie madness and distress, and onto the individual, as opposed to collective forms of support.

With this in mind, how do service users, survivors, activists and mental health professionals ensure that recovery retains its radical roots and guarantee that those with lived experience of madness and distress are the authors and arbiters of their own recovery stories? In this important book, which will be of tremendous use to those with self-experience, a general audience and for all practitioners, Mike Watts and Agnes Higgins, along with their 26 expert-by-experience collaborators, provide an invaluable exploration of these tensions. Crucially, they advocate the importance of finding creative ways to resist the constraining effects of the clinical gaze one is subject to during and beyond psychiatric treatment and demonstrate that collective action and peer support are central to an empowered and truly transformational process of recovery.

Jacqui Dillon,
Chair, National Hearing Voices Network, England
London, 2016

Acknowledgements

We the authors would like to acknowledge first and foremost the contribution made by the 26 members of GROW in Ireland whose stories of recovery from 'mental illness' have illuminated the pages of this book. Their rich and generous narratives, we believe, will represent a real beacon of hope to other people struggling with their mental health and searching to find a road to recovery. These stories are also an invaluable source of information for mental health professionals and family members whose aim is to support people in their recovery and who have the potential to improve the quality of mental health care.

We would like to extend a sincere thank-you to the following:

Carol Mussey, International Program Coordinator, GROW International, and Jacqui Dillon, Chair, National Hearing Voices Network, England, for taking the time to write forewords.

Angela Kendrick, John Kidney, John Rice and Margaret Williams, who painstakingly provided feedback on the way in which we have presented the book's findings.

Carmel Downes, Sonam Prakashini Banka and Lorna Higgins for their help with the administrative aspect of preparing the book and their meticulous attention to referencing.

Peter Dabinett of Kilkenny Design Consultancy for his work on Making a Recovery Map.

We would also like to thank the management of GROW in Ireland and the School of Nursing and Midwifery in Trinity College Dublin, Ireland, and the countless people in the recovery movement who kept us motivated by continuously enquiring about our progress.

A thank-you to Clare Ashworth, Emily Bedford, Jane Madeley and Thomas Storr at Routledge Books for their patience and timely advice throughout the whole writing and production process.

Finally a huge thank-you to Fran Watts and James P. O'Neill, our spouses, who witnessed and supported us in the ups and downs involved in bringing this book into being.

Thank you: Peter, Tom, Kate, Jess, Mags, Jack, James, Paul, Mathew, Nan, Sue, Charlie, Peg, Ruth, David, Helen, Penny, Vicky, Martha, Pat, Frances, Danny, Richard, Cathy, Lynn and Claire. May you remain re-enchanted by life.

1   Genesis of the book and setting the context

The word 'recovery' from mental health problems is 'in the air'. Everyone is talking about it. Go to any mental health website, sit in on any mental health services development meeting, scan through the curriculum of any education programme for mental health professionals and the word 'recovery' is going to be found. Everyone is asking 'Is this service recovery oriented?', 'Is this education programme underpinned by recovery values?'; and the likelihood is that everyone will nod in the affirmative, looking somewhat affronted that the question should be asked in the first place. Is that not what the whole mental health system is about?

Since the 1990s many Western governments have announced policies that champion the idea of recovery. For example, America *'envisions a future when everyone with a mental illness will recover'* (President's New Freedom Commission on Mental Health 2003:1). Similarly New Zealand's publication 'Recovery Competencies for New Zealand Mental Health Workers' (Mental Health Commission New Zealand 2001) and the UK's policy document 'The Journey to Recovery – The Government's Vision for Mental Health Care' (Department of Health 2001) all seek to make recovery the main aim of their mental health systems. In Ireland with the publication of 'A Vision for Change: Report of the Expert Group on Mental Health Policy' (Department of Health and Children 2006) the government articulated a commitment to transforming mental health services to recovery-oriented principles. Despite growth in the usage of the word 'recovery' within policy and practice discourse, very legitimate questions remain. What does recovery from 'mental illness' mean? How is it achieved and how can it be nurtured? Is it a chemical process or a learning and developmental journey? Is serious 'mental illness' a permanent condition that requires life-long treatment, or is it indicative of an emotional crisis that is fully resolvable?

The word 'recovery' is packed with multiple meanings. Any English dictionary might define recovery as an action or process of regaining possession or control of something stolen or lost or, in a health context, describe it as a return to a normal state of health, mind or strength. Deegan (1995), a mental health activist with self-experience of mental health problems, views recovery as a process through which people acknowledge being socially disabled by their mental health problems and recover a new sense of self. Anthony (1993:527) developed these ideas further by contending that '*recovery involved the development of new meaning and purpose in one's life as one grows beyond the catastrophic effects of mental illness*'. This means moving away from the currently dominant idea that recovery is primarily to do with a medically supervised process involving medications, the removal of 'symptoms' of illness or the return to some 'pre-illness' state.

Shari McDaid (2013:8), the CEO of Ireland's Mental Health Reform, describes recovery as an

> individual process of discovering one's own strengths, values, meaning and aspirations; a self-determined journey that can take place inside and outside the mental health system, through personal development, through partnership relationships with professionals, through peer support or through community support.

It is a process of reconnecting with life that can happen for some with the continuation of 'symptoms', while for others, a reduction in 'symptoms' is important. This view challenges the idea that recovery from mental distress or 'mental illness' must take place within the boundaries of traditional mental health services and is solely dependent on the support of mental health professionals. McDaid's (2013) view opens up the potential for mental health problems to be resolved within the context of the social system, within the day-to-day interactions people have within their communities and through peer and community support.

This book is largely about recovery from 'mental illness' outside the boundaries of traditional mental health services. It is a story of possibility and hope involving the recovery stories of people, all of whom received a diagnosis of 'mental illness' and all of whom were involved in mutual support through an organisation known as GROW. What emerges from their stories is a powerful and fantastic story of human effort and healing. This book also tells a story of the capacity for mutual or peer support to reach into the most hidden recesses of human experience and enable a person to find strength, personal meaning and identity. While individual accounts highlight many of the deficiencies of a mental health system rooted in the idea that 'mental illness' is symptomatic of a problem within the person, be it genetic or chemical, there is an acknowledgement that medical treatment can, when implemented in dialogue with the person, be an invaluable start to the recovery journey. However, there is also a strong suggestion that recovery can include an appropriate weaning away from the need for medication as other personal, inter-personal and social resources are developed and put into place.

While the two people named on the cover of this book, Mike Watts and Agnes Higgins, are the official authors, in fact the real authors of this book consist of the 26 people interviewed about their experiences and journeys. They are the people who put the words on the pages, and we (Mike and Agnes) could be viewed as merely the pen which gave their stories flesh. Having said this, our own biographies no doubt have shaped our interest in the subject area and our chosen method of collecting and analysing the stories. We both have spent our entire adult lives connected in different ways to the field of mental health and during that time have struggled with the meaning of the concept of recovery, including how best to support and nurture it. Both of us have been close observers of the way people diagnosed with 'mental illness' have been treated and the effects this treatment has had on them. In different ways we both have been at the very center of Ireland's own efforts to develop a recovery ethos, Mike through his own personal experience of 'mental illness' and recovery and his peer-support work and Agnes through her experience of working as a nurse within the formal mental health services and hospice services and through her research and teaching in the area of mental health.

Mike and Agnes first met in the early 2000s, when Mike came to co-facilitate some teaching sessions on recovery for student mental health nurses with Agnes in Trinity College Dublin, Ireland. Later, as Mike went on to read for a PhD, Agnes became his mentor and academic supervisor. Since then they have collaborated on a number of projects and initiatives, including this book. In keeping with the spirit of the book and in an attempt not to mirror or add to the disparities of power within what is termed the 'service user/professional relationship', they would like to tell you something about their lives and motivations so that they are not just anonymous names with academic titles and qualifications.

Something about Mike

I grew up in a medical family. Both my parents were doctors, and my father's special interest was mental illness in general practice. As a young man I became increasingly beset by fears about myself, about life and about the future. These were exacerbated by a growing reliance on alcohol and later cannabis. On occasion, I had begun to hear menacing voices and to misinterpret the meaning of everyday sounds. I had also begun to develop theories about eye colour that I knew were very strange, and yet I resisted seeking help. Towards the end of the 1960s I agreed to see a psychiatrist, a friend of my father. I thought I was headed for a quiet personal chat where I would find reassurance and perhaps some guidance on how I could help myself. Instead, I was asked if medical students could sit in on my first interview. I can still picture a whole group of them in a small lecture theatre with eager faces and notebooks. I could feel myself clamming shut and wanting to escape. After the interview I was given a diagnosis of pathological shyness, prescribed Librium and told that I was welcome to come back whenever I liked. I never did go back. In 1973, after the birth of our first child, my wife Fran experienced what was termed a classic post-puerperal psychosis. It was probably the most frightening experience of both of our lives. Admitted to hospital and treated solely with drugs, Fran's diagnoses oscillated between schizophrenia, schizo-affective disorder and bipolar or manic depression. Nobody could offer any advice on how we could help ourselves other than to 'keep on taking the tablets'. No one ever asked us about ourselves or about any of the traumas we had both experienced along the way. The blunt manner with which Fran was told she had schizophrenia completely stole any hope she might have for the future. She was told that she would need lifelong medication and frequent respite breaks in hospital and should avoid all kinds of stress. The side effects of the medication were horrendous. Fran's life was over. Barely able to function and massively overweight, we were both told 'you are cured', go and get on with your life.

Those two incidents formed the basis of a lifelong passionate interest in recovery. In 1976 we stumbled across GROW, a mutual-help organisation working in the area of mental health. It was manna from heaven. Through GROW we met people who supported us in our recovery, and we, in return, mutually supported them. After 7 years of voluntary involvement with GROW I became a fieldworker and then national program coordinator, a role I played for 20 years.

As part of my own recovery I returned to third-level study, studying psychology and later family therapy. I also became involved in many artistic groups such as painting, writing, music and poetry. In the mid 2000s, at the end of a 5-year spell as a service user member of Ireland's newly formed Mental Health Commission and after spending more than 30 years working in the area of recovery, I undertook a PhD degree.

Something about Agnes

I grew up in the west of Ireland, a middle child of seven, two sisters and a brother older and two sisters and a brother younger. Born into a small rural farming community, I was no stranger to farm work and the long idyllic days in the hay field or bog, but neither was I a stranger to the harshness of rural communities when one was perceived as different. The stigma and shame associated with having a 'mental illness' or having to spend time in the local psychiatric institution was very real, with very real consequences for the person and family concerned.

I commenced mental health nurse training in 1978, not exactly with the approval of my parents, as they worried about me and would have preferred if I had chosen 'real nursing' (general nursing). Indeed, I am still unsure why I chose mental health nursing. My decision to accept a place as a student psychiatric nurse, in St Vincent's Hospital Fairview, Dublin, Ireland, was strongly influenced by the warm, friendly and caring atmosphere created by the people who interviewed me. Some might say it was a naive way to make a decision about something as serious as my future career. Looking back, I feel fortunate as I have never known a morning that I was not excited or hopeful about going in to work, whether I was working in a mental health service, hospice, general hospital or an academic institution. This is not to suggest that I was not challenged or distressed by the stories I heard, the people I met or the inadequacies of the services and system that I was part of and, some might even say, supported and maintained.

Early in my career in mental health I was fortunate to be introduced to the writings of Ervin Goffman (1959, 1961, 1963) by one of my tutors and later given a copy of Peter Breggin's (1991) book *Toxic Psychiatry*. Reading these authors was a transformative experience and no doubt shaped the way I now think about mental distress and the supports we offer people at their most vulnerable. Reading these books also put me at odds with the prevailing 'medical wisdom' at the time and set me on my own journey of discovery and recovery, which I am still on.

Although I have been challenged in so many ways in my life, I have enjoyed the privilege of what I would term good mental health, but like so many, I have encountered the distress of mental health problems within my close family and friends. Together, my family members, friends and the people that I met within the mental health services have challenged me to strip away the arrogance of the 'professional', and in doing so they have taught me the importance of revealing my own vulnerabilities and humanity. I am indebted to them all for affording me the possibility of getting to know the essence of their being and in the process to get to know myself better.

Something about the use of language

Language is not just a neutral vehicle for expressing our thoughts, emotions and desires in everyday social interaction. It has the potential to shape our thoughts and behaviours, restrict or expand our understanding and conceptualization of the world. Similarly, the language used throughout this book has the potential to narrowly frame thinking or be seen as an expression of 'solidarity' with a particular world view. Hence, there is a need for some comment on the debate around the socially constructed nature of terms such as 'mental illness' and 'mental disorder'. While the most appropriate term for and the real nature of 'mental illness' are hotly debated issues within the literature, the term 'mental illness' currently remains the most widely used description in both professional and lay conversations. Even though 'mental illness' is a term that is considered medically laden it is used in this book, alongside 'mental distress', for a number of reasons. GROW, the organisation whose members told their stories, use the term 'mental illness' in their literature (GROW 2001:24) even though they take issue with the medical interpretation of this phrase, and many of the people interviewed used the term. Indeed, by being so medically laden the words 'mental illness' may reflect the growing body of opinion that recovery from 'mental illness' also implicitly includes recovery from a system that relies too heavily on a medical explanation of distress.

We also use the word *stories* rather than discourses, dialogues or perspectives because the method used to explore people's experience of recovery was an approach which invited people to tell their own spontaneous personal story at a particular moment in time and within the 'space' of an interview. Subsuming these experiential accounts under the rubric of 'story' hopefully serves to elevate the value of knowledge forged through lived experience, and indicates our belief that personal stories based on an experience of 'mental illness', treatment and recovery need to be added to the traditional hierarchies of professionally authoritative knowledge and evidence that underpin mental health practice.

Something about the book

This book has been written with a wide range of people in mind, including those with self-experience of 'mental illness' or distress, those supporting them informally through peer support and family, friends and significant others. It also has something to say to those who formally support people through traditional mental health services, such as practitioners working in the field of mental health from an array of disciplines, including medicine, nursing, social work, occupational therapy or psychology. In addition, we hope the book will appeal to those who may not have direct experience of mental distress but who are interested in learning more.

The book has two main aims. The first is to tell the story of people's journeys from places of severe mental distress and despair to places of recovery, and their journey to a discovery of meaning and purpose in self and in life, beyond diagnosis. The second is to give the reader insight into how vital mutual help and mutual support can be in people's recovery journeys. We hope that the book will act as a point of hope and inspiration for people who are struggling with 'mental illness' or distress and will help them discover their own path towards recovery. We hope that it will help people working within the boundaries of traditional mental health services appreciate the potential role of mutual help in people's recovery journeys and consider ways they might begin collaborating with peer-support services, not just as an 'alternative' other but as a fundamental part of the service offered to people in a manner that complements current services. We also hope that the book will be a fitting tribute and thank-you to the 26 people who told us their story. Overall, we hope that the book will provide an alternative way of looking at 'mental illness' or distress and demonstrate that there are many relatively unexplored avenues and paths to recovery that need to be considered.

Section 1 of this book begins with an overview of the two dominant stories about mental distress and 'mental illness' that tend to shape our understanding: namely the biomedical and rehabilitation story. This is followed by a chapter that explores the current emergence of the recovery story, its meaning and the evidence underpinning this story. As the focus of the book is on recovery stories through mutual help, the meaning, origins, reported benefits and weaknesses of mutual help is the subject of another chapter, which is written in the context of a discussion on GROW, the mutual-support group used by the people that are the focus of this book. Section 1 of the book concludes with an exploration of how the study was conducted and describes the narrative methodology employed within this study.

Section 2, the heart of the book, presents the findings of the study, which collectively represents the stories of the 26 people interviewed and depicts recovery as a 're-enchantment with life'. Recovery, as a re-enchantment with life, is portrayed as an ongoing process of personal empowerment and liberation through reciprocal and healing involvement with others. People described becoming re-enchanted by new and exciting ideas about themselves, about others and about the future which were initially triggered by encounters with the hopeful culture of mutual support. People described how they escaped from the alienated isolation of 'mental illness' through participation in the small, compassionate social body of a weekly mutual-support group. During this 'time of healing' unexpected feelings of hope, joy and belonging spawned new and exciting ways of thinking and relating to others, so that over time people began to gather the spiritual ingredients of resilience.

Recovery involved a successful re-integration into society through involvements in carefully chosen niches of employment, education and leisure. Recovery and re-enchantment were confirmed as people assumed positive social identities and realised their radical equality with others, the value of their own suffering and that they could choose a future that would enhance and maintain an exciting, meaningful and fulfilling life.

Being mindful that the book will be read by academics, researchers and policy makers, Section 3, the conclusion, reviews and revisits eight core processes that were central to people's recovery in order to discuss, theorise and highlight how and why these processes enabled each person deal successfully with life, even when life became extremely difficult. In addition a number of diagrams developed from our conceptualisation of the recovery process and which may be used to open discussion about recovery are also included. The book concludes with a discussion on the implications of the research for an emerging model of a recovery-oriented mental health service.

In conclusion, Repper and Perkins (2003), both people who openly acknowledged their self-experience of 'mental illness', suggest that the word 'recovery' should perhaps be replaced with the word 'discovery'. We hope that your journey through this book will be a journey of discovery, not just about the people within the book but a journey of discovery about yourself and your own mental health.

References

Anthony, W. A. 1993. Recovery from mental illness: The guiding vision of the mental health service system in the 1990s. *Psychosocial Rehabilitation Journal*, 16, 521–537.

Breggin, P. R. 1991. *Toxic psychiatry*, New York, St. Martin's Press.

Deegan, P. 1995. Coping with recovery as a journey of the heart. *Psychiatric Rehabilitation Journal*, 19, 91–97.

Department of Health 2001. *The journey to recovery: The government's vision for mental health care*, London, Department of Health.

Department of Health and Children 2006. *A vision for change: Report of the expert group on mental health policy*, Dublin, Stationery Office.

Goffman, E. 1959. *The presentation of self in everyday life*, London, Penguin Books.

Goffman, E. 1961. *Asylums: Essays on the social situations of mental patients and other inmates*, New York, Anchor.

Goffman, E. 1963. *Stigma: Notes on the management of spoiled identity*, New York, Simon and Schuster.

GROW 2001. *Program of growth maturity*, Sydney, GROW Publications.

McDaid, S. 2013. *Recovery: What you should expect from a good quality mental health service*, Dublin, Mental Health Reform.

Mental Health Commission 2001. *Recovery competencies for New Zealand mental health workers*, Wellington, New Zealand, Mental health Commission.

President's New Freedom Commission on Mental Health 2003. *Achieving the promise: Transforming mental health care in America*, Rockville, MD, DHHS.

Repper, J. & Perkins, R. 2003. *Social inclusion and recovery: A model for mental health practice*, London, Baillière Tindall.

2 The medicalisation of human distress

> There is a difference between knowledge and wisdom. . . . For example when we teach our students about the heart we teach them that the heart is a pump; a type of organic machine with valves and chambers. And indeed, in time they learn to recognize the anatomical heart in all its detail. After passing their final anatomy exam we say, 'This student knows about the heart'. But in wisdom we would have to doubt this statement. Wisdom would seek the form or the essence of the heart. It would have us understand that there is another heart; the heart that can break; the heart that grows weary; the heart that leaps with joy; the one that lives in my body and in your body.
>
> (Deegan 1995:91)

We live within a world of 'made-up' stories, and these stories impose some kind of order upon the world and help us deal with reality (Frank 1995, Rappaport 2000, Bruner 2002). Throughout history mankind has created stories seeking to explain the phenomenon of 'mental illness' or 'emotional distress', suggesting various explanations around meaning and cause and giving rise to a range of strategies and processes to facilitate its amelioration. As Deegan (1995:91) suggests in the opening quote, many of these stories fail to adequately grasp the complexity of the human being.

The medical story of 'mental illness' is a story which has undergone a number of transformations while retaining many constant identifiable characteristics. Having wrestled control of 'lunatic' asylums from lay administrators, psychiatry sought to tame 'madness' and gain credibility by aligning itself with mainstream medicine. Bracken *et al.* (2012:430) argue that throughout the 19th and 20th centuries,

> psychiatry held fast to the idea that mental health problems are best understood through a biomedical idiom; that problems with feelings, thoughts, behaviours, and relationships can be fully grasped with the sort of scientific tools that we use to investigate problems with our livers and lungs.

Drawing on positivist ideologies and aligned with scientific principles as applied to the physical body, the medical story of psychiatry postulated that mental health problems and mental distress are a form of 'illness' that can be objectively observed, measured, verified and controlled through the study of the brain, its biochemical interactions, its neurons and each person's genetic constitution. Within this perspective mental health problems are viewed as internal to the individual and primarily due to some faulty physiological or psychological mechanism. The meaning people attach to their experience of mental distress is not considered relevant and is more or less ignored. Commentators on the biomedical story note that each newly 'discovered' theory and its accompanying treatment has been heralded as a 'major scientific advance', while negative outcomes have been excluded or at best minimised (Scull 1979, Breggin 1991, Johnstone 2000). Others suggest that while purporting to be 'objective', the theories put forward within the medical story have been greatly influenced by the personal views of each emerging theorist and the political, social and economic ideas of the time (Whitaker 2010).

Early medical stories and claims about mental illness

Thomas Willis (1648) is accredited with being the first person to construct a medical paradigm of 'mental illness' (Whitaker 2002). Philosophies of the time had concluded that man was 'separated from the beast' through the faculty of reason, and in this context, Willis proposed that insanity was caused by a loss of reason. Its cure lay in the restoration of reason through professionally administered 'tortures and torments'. In Willis's words: 'maniacs often recover much sooner, if they are treated with tortures and torments in a hovel instead of with medicaments' (Willis 1684 cited in Whitaker 2002:6). And so the stage was set for a whole range of theories and practices that were advanced and practised by a branch of medicine that, Scull (1979) speculates, was desperate to gain academic credibility. Treatments included spinning chairs, prolonged immersion in baths, exposure to extremes of temperature, injections of a wide variety of substances, purges and of course restraint through the use of chains (Scull 1979, Johnstone 2000, Whitaker 2002). Henry Cotton (1919), no doubt influenced by advances in mainstream medicine and by the successful cure of syphilitic paresis, speculated that insanity must be caused by bacterial infection of the brain. The most obvious cure therefore was the removal of the seat of infection, first through tooth extraction, then tonsils and then parts of the bowels. Cotton's work was recently described in the *Lancet* as 'a tale of such gothic horror that the author must assure his readers the events he recounts really happened' (Hudson Jones 2005:361). Despite this, 'when the fallacies of Cotton's claims and the harms of his treatments had been investigated and reported by other psychiatrists, their reports were disregarded or suppressed' (Hudson Jones 2005:362). Psychiatry confidently marched on, with a whole new batch of what was considered revolutionary treatments, including insulin and malarial coma treatment, lobotomy and metrazole convulsive therapy, the forerunner to today's electro-convulsive therapy. All of these were believed to work on various parts of the brain, the site and cause of 'mental illness', all were hailed as 'miracle therapies', achieving academic and practical dominance, and all damaging lives while making claims about positive outcomes (Whitaker 2002, 2010, Healy 2004). Indeed, Egas Moniz, the neurosurgeon who introduced frontal lobotomies, received the Nobel Prize for Medicine in 1949.

The eugenics story

The eugenics[1] movement, which was strongly influenced by Darwin's work on evolutionary theory, and Spencer and Galton's theory on inheritance and moral degeneracy had followers within psychiatry (Shorter 1997). The eugenics movement argued that mental distress was caused by 'bad brain plasma' or 'cacogenic genes' (Davenport 1911:241); consequently, eminent psychiatrists began to see insanity as the end stage of a family's germ plasm deterioration: 'The insane patient gets it from where his parents got it – from the insane strain of the family stock' (Maudsley 1895 cited in Whitaker 2002:45).

Premised on the belief that 'mental illness' had a strong genetic component and procreation among people with mental health problems would lead to social degeneracy and 'race suicide', social hygienists campaigned for restrictions on people's right to reproduce (Shorter 1997). Adherents to the eugenics movement frequently cited evidence that people with 'mental illness' were hypersexual, immoral and governed by animalistic sexual urges (Whitaker 2002). This resulted in mass segregation of those deemed 'insane' and the introduction of enforced sterilisation programmes. In 1935 Nobel-winning physician Alexis Carrel gave voice to the idea that the 'insane' 'should be humanely and economically disposed of in small euthanasic institutions supplied with proper gases' (Carrel 1935:318). By 1914 eugenics was being taught in 44 American colleges of psychiatry, and by 1924, 9,000 papers had been printed on the subject (Whitaker 2002:53). A travelling show titled 'Some People are Born to be a Burden on the Rest' toured America, educating the general public. Nazi Germany and the Second World War gave rise to the full horrors and implications of eugenic thinking. Hitler's 1933 sterilisation bill was seen by American psychiatrists as a public endorsement of the value of their work: 'The leaders in the German sterilisation movement repeatedly state that their legislation was formulated only after careful study of the California experiments' (Smyth 1938 cited in Whitaker 2002:63).

Within Ireland, Connolly Norman, a leading Irish psychiatrist in the early 1900s, presented what he considered proof that 'feeble-minded' people produced larger families than did 'sound-minded' people (Nolan 1993:38). Supporters of the eugenics movement often referred their British audience to the position in Ireland where, they claimed, hundreds of 'defectives' were being allowed to reproduce, leading to degeneracy on a large scale (Nolan 1993:38). Shorter (1997) suggests that it was only after the atrocities of World War II that the degeneracy theory and reference to eugenics became a social and professional taboo. Although degeneracy theory has been discounted within the scientific literature, people with mental health problems having children continues to be met with disapproval within Irish society (National Disability Authority 2011).

The classification and categorisation of distress stories

The classification story of 'mental illness' came in the form of a categorisation system that described mental distress as a collection of illnesses and diagnoses, each with its own collection of symptoms and signs. The origin of this system is generally accepted as evolving from Emile Kraepelin, who in 1887 described the medical condition 'dementia praecox', a brain condition that led to a sustained state of madness. MacGabhann (2014:28) suggests that 'although the initial classifications were purported to be "physical" or observable biological symptoms of brain dysfunction, they were generally not physically observable or indeed related to obvious biological function'. Nonetheless, psychiatry laid claim to a classification framework, with those who came after adding to and elaborating on the framework. Today we have two recognised classification systems: the WHO's *International Classifications of Diseases* (ICD) and the American Psychiatric Association's *Diagnosis and Statistical Manual of Mental Disorders* (DSM) and their subsequent editions. Within this system each diagnosis is defined by a list of symptoms, with a numerical threshold that must be achieved in the symptoms before a diagnosis can be made (Angell 2011). Having commenced in 1952 with 106 diagnoses, today the DSM classification system provides a technical reference point for defining more than 360 'mental illnesses'. While the main goal of each classification system is to bring consistency or diagnostic reliability among clinicians and researchers, especially in a world of increasing pharmacological treatments, critics argue that while diagnostic criteria may provide a set of 'symptoms and signs' that enable researchers to achieve inter-rater reliability, diagnostic labels wrench ownership of the experience from the person, thus denying their own attempt to make sense of the experience, and do little to help our understanding of the inner world of the person (Rappaport 2000). Others raise questions around diagnostic validity or factual soundness (Rosenhan 1973, Lynch 2001, Whitaker 2002), viewing the diagnostic process as a deeply flawed system that ignores and masks gender, racial and cultural bias (Kleinman 1988, Charon 2006). Kutchins and Kirk (1997:28) commenting on the validity of the DSM, contend that it

> is a book of tentatively assembled agreements. . . . You can have agreements among experts without validity. Even if you found four people who agreed that the earth is flat, the moon is made of cheese, that smoking cigarettes poses no health risks, or that politicians are never corrupt, such agreements do not establish truth.

Although some people are happy to define the mental distress and problems experienced by others using a biomedical classification, many others, for various reasons, reject the whole diagnostic framework. Some reject it on the ground that the language of psychopathology is oppressive and does not speak to a person's individual distress. Others comment on the loss of identity that often accompanies a diagnosis, as the diagnostic label subsumes all other identities (Deegan 1995, Fisher 2005), becoming the person's primary identity or 'master status' (Goffman 1963).

The pharmacological story

The biochemical or pharmacology story, the current dominant and authoritative medical story, heralds 'an age characterised by the idea that drugs can cure mental illness' (Moncrieff 2007:1). The pharmacological story of 'mental illness' is based on the premise that 'mental illness' is related to some biochemical or biological malfunction within the brain (Hoff 2008); thus drugs can work on specific areas of the brain, changing biochemical balances and thus restoring mental health. Shorter, commenting on the introduction of the new 'wonder drug' chlorpromazine to the American market in May 1954, summed up this belief: 'Chlorpromazine initiated a revolution in psychiatry, comparable to the introduction of penicillin in general medicine . . . Ensuring for the first time, that schizophrenic patients could lead relatively normal lives and not be confined in institutions' (Shorter 1997:255).

Theories explaining the aetiology of 'mental illness' in terms of serotonin and dopamine levels are now central to the academic training of psychiatrists and other mental health practitioners and, through them, the general public. When viewed in the context of previous medical stories, one has to ask how much of the thinking behind the pharmacological story is 'fact' and how much is imagination or market propaganda. People are told that these drugs counter a chemical imbalance in much the same way as insulin treats diabetes and, like insulin, drugs will be required for life if not for an extended period of time. Yet there is limited evidence to support the biochemical theory, and unlike diabetes, no test exists to measure serotonin or dopamine deficiency or excess (Breggin 1991, Lynch 2001, Healy 2004). People are also told that the closure of the large institutions was largely due to the introduction of pharmacology, which controlled 'symptoms', enabling people to live in the community; yet detailed analysis suggests that deinstitutionalisation came about as the result of economic and social imperatives, combined with the realisation of the negative impact of institutionalisation (Brennan 2014).

While many people report benefits from drug treatments, how these benefits come about is still largely unclear. Some studies suggest that long-term outcomes for people with a diagnosis of schizophrenia who are not treated with psychiatric drugs are far better than for people who are treated with drugs (Mosher and Menn 1970, World Health Organisation (WHO) 1979, Harding *et al.* 1987, Harrison *et al.* 2001). There is also a growing awareness of harmful side effects including parkinsonism, tardive dyskinesia, hypotension, sexual dysfunction, weight gain, diabetes mellitus and neuroleptic malignant syndrome (Slade 2009, Higgins *et al.* 2010). Questions have also been raised about relationships among drug companies, academic psychiatry and researchers, with a growing critique of the manner in which negative outcomes of drug trials are supressed, generating biased evidence (Whitaker 2010, Healy 2012). It is not surprising that Rappaport (2005) believes that an 'unholy alliance' has been formed between science and state, an alliance that has sacrificed human values in a mad rush for prestige, profit and power. Despite all the question marks about the pharmacological story, for the majority of people drug therapy remains the treatment of choice by many mental health practitioners and the primary form of help offered to people seeking relief from 'mental distress'. In Ireland, as elsewhere, the demands for antidepressants, tranquillisers and other drugs used within psychiatry is exponentially on the increase (Department of Health and Children 2006, Dunne 2006, Feldman *et al.* 2006).

The rehabilitation story

The 'rehabilitation' or the 'psychosocial rehabilitation' story, emerged in the 1960s and 1970s with the aim of helping people leave behind institutional care and enable those diagnosed with 'chronic mental illness' to integrate into the community and live independently. Rössler (2006:151) states the goal of 'psychiatric rehabilitation is to help individuals with persistent and serious mental illness to develop the emotional, social and intellectual skills needed to live, learn and work in the community with the least amount of professional support'. Although sometimes spoken of as different to the medical model, the rehabilitation story is largely based on the medical view, assuming that mental distress is an 'illness', similar to a spinal injury. While the injury itself can never be cured, with rehabilitation, a person can find 'some semblance of the life they had before the illness' (Andresen *et al.* 2003:588). Similar to other medical stories, the rehabilitation story is an ascribed hierarchy (Kloos 1999). The skills required of the person experiencing mental distress are objectively defined and assessed by the 'expert professional', and the care and treatment provided occur within the confines of day hospitals, day centers, sheltered employment and community residences or hostels. While rehabilitation services are considered by some to predict better longitudinal outcomes for serious 'mental illness' (DeSisto *et al.* 1995), others, including former service user and advocate Patricia Deegan, take issue with the oppressive connotations of the term 'rehabilitation', arguing that people are not passive objects to be rehabilitated but active agents in their own change process. She is also of the view that many rehabilitation programmes simply cultivate a different form of institutionalisation, with people becoming trapped in what she terms 'desolate wastelands of mental health programmes' (Deegan 1995:3). Rappaport (1998) suggests that once a rehabilitation programme, however good it may be, comes to an end, then progress made within that programme is habitually reversed.

Ireland's mental health services are perhaps no different to those of other countries which claim to have progressed along the lines of rehabilitation and community integration. In McDaid's (2014) view, these moves, instead of signalling the personal liberation and recovery of people who had been institutionalised, have resulted in a re-institutionalisation of people within the community. Drawing on numerous reports and research studies published throughout the 1990s and 2000s, she concludes that findings from these

> put paid to any idea that individuals living in mental health service-staffed accommodation were living deinstitutionalised lives' as their lives in the residences were still highly institutional, while their lives outside of the residences were largely confined to mental health service–related activities.
>
> (McDaid 2014:51)

Similar conclusions were reached about those attending day services, with McDaid (2014:51) commenting that people were 'trapped in mental health day services with little opportunity for integration in the community'. While the rehabilitation model may have espoused community integration, and people may have moved to reside in the community, they do not appear to be living integrated lives within that community. In many cases, people are trapped in mini institutions and have merely traded one form of institutional oppression for another, this time modelled on a rehabilitation story.

Concluding comments

The medical story of 'mental illness' views mental distress as an essential component of a person's biological makeup. Consequently, there is a search for 'truth' within the structure and function of the physical body. Within this reductionist view, biology is considered the dominant source of illness, with people experiencing mental distress studied as 'objects' or clinical entities and where the meaning associated with their experience and life contexts is ignored, minimised or not considered relevant.

While the 'scientific method' does bring benefits in the form of new inventions and interventions in health care, in the area of human experience and mental distress, it does have limitations and only provides part of the story. Human beings are not just physical objects, devoid of agency, choice, reason and sense-making potential; they actively engage with, interpret and respond to the world. In addition, generalisable information generated from large groups does not illuminate individual processes or experiences or the meaning different individuals attach to those experiences. Slade (2009:10) is of the view that filtering human experience through the medical or psychopathological sieve results in an impoverished and decontextualized version of meaning.

In addition, the story of 'mental illness' produced through this method tends to dominate all other stories, and as writers such as Kuhn (1962) and Foucault (2001) point out, in the battle for political supremacy, it is authority, and in this case medical authority, that dictates which stories are believed, which stories hold the greatest power and which stories get subjugated or marginalised.

Note

1 In 1883 Galton coined the term 'eugenics', derived from the Greek word for 'well born', as a name for a science devoted to improving the human race (Whitaker 2002).

References

Andresen, R., Oades, L. & Caputi, P. 2003. The experience of recovery from schizophrenia: Towards an empirically validated stage model. *Australian and New Zealand Journal of Psychiatry*, 37, 586–594.

Angell, M. 2011. The illusions of psychiatry. *The New York Review*, July 14th.

Bracken, P., Thomas, P., Timimi, S., Asen, E., Behr, G., Beuster, C., Bhunnoo, S., Browne, I., Chhina, N., Double, D., Downer, S., Evans, C., Fernando, S., Garland, M. R., Hopkins, W., Huws, R., Johnson, B., Martindale, B., Middleton, H., Moldavsky, D., Moncrieff, J., Mullins, S., Nelki, J., Pizzo, M., Rodger, J., Smyth, M., Summerfield, D., Wallace, J. & Yeomans, D. 2012. Psychiatry beyond the current paradigm. *The British Journal of Psychiatry*, 201, 430–434.

Breggin, P. R. 1991. *Toxic psychiatry*, New York, St. Martin's Press.

Brennan, D. 2014. *Irish insanity 1800–2000: Routledge advances in sociology*, Oxon, Routledge.

Bruner, J. 2002. *Making stories: Law, literature, life*, Cambridge, MA, London, Harvard University Press.

Carrel, A. 1935. *Man, the unknown*, New York, Penguin.

Charon, R. 2006. *Narrative medicine: Honoring the stories of illness*, Oxford, Oxford University Press.

Cotton, H. 1919. The relation of oral infection to mental diseases. *Journal of Dental Research*, 1, 269–313.

Davenport, C. B. 1911. *Heredity in relation to eugenics*, New York, Henry Holt.

Deegan, P. 1995. Coping with recovery as a journey of the heart. *Psychiatric Rehabilitation Journal*, 19, 91–97.

Department of Health and Children 2006. *A vision for change: Report of the expert group on mental health policy*, Dublin, Stationery Office.

Desisto, M. J., Harding, C. M., McCormick, R. V., Ashikaga, T. & Brooks, G. W. 1995. The Maine and Vermont three-decade studies of serious mental illness. II. Matched comparison of cross-sectional. Longitudinal course comparisons. *The British Journal of Psychiatry*, 167, 338–342.

Dunne, E. 2006. *The views of adult users of the public sector mental health services*, Dublin, Ireland, Mental Health Commission.

Feldman, M. D., Franks, P., Epstein, R. M., Franz, C. E. & Kravitz, R. L. 2006. Do patient requests for antidepressants enhance or hinder physicians' evaluation of depression? A randomized controlled trial. *Medical Care*, 44, 1107–1113.

Fisher, D. 2005. An empowerment model of recovery from severe mental illness: An expert interview. *Medscape Psychiatry & Mental Health*, 10, 1–5.

Foucault, M. 2001. Power/knowledge. *In*: Seidman, S. & Alexander, Jeffrey C. (eds.) *The new social theory reader: Contemporary debates* (pp. 69–75), New York, Routledge.

Frank, A. 1995. *The wounded storyteller: Body, illness, and ethics*, Chicago, University of Chicago Press.

Goffman, E. 1963. *Stigma: Notes on the management of spoiled identity*, New York, Simon and Schuster.

Harding, C. M., Brooks, G., Ashikaga, T., Strauss, J. & Breier, A. 1987. The Vermont longitudinal study of persons with severe mental illness. *American Journal of Community Psychiatry*, 144, 718–735.

Harrison, G., Hopper, K., Craig, T., Laska, E., Siegel, C., Wanderling, J., Dube, K., Ganev, K., Giel, R. & Der Heiden, W. A. 2001. Recovery from psychotic illness: A 15-and 25-year international follow-up study. *The British Journal of Psychiatry*, 178, 506–517.

Healy, D. 2004. *Let them eat Prozac: The unhealthy relationship between the pharmaceutical companies and depression*, New York, New York University.

Healy, D. 2012. *Pharmageddon*, Berkeley, University of California Press.

Higgins, A., Nash, M. & Lynch, A. M. 2010. Antidepressant-associated sexual dysfunction: Impact, effects, and treatment. *Drug, Healthcare and Patient Safety*, 2, 141–150.

Hoff, P. 2008. Kraeplin and degeneration theory. *European Archives of Psychiatry and Clinical Neuroscience*, 258, 12–17.

Hudson Jones, A. 2005. The cautionary tale of psychiatrist Henry Aloysius Cotton. *The Lancet*, 366, 361–362.

Johnstone, L. 2000. *Users and abusers of psychiatry: A critical look at psychiatric practice*, New York, Routledge.

Kleinman, A. 1988. *The illness narratives: Suffering, healing, and the human condition*, New York, Basic Books.

Kloos, B. 1999. *Cultivating identity: Meaning making in the context of residential treatment settings for persons with histories of psychological disorders*. Unpublished doctoral dissertation, University of Illinois at Urbana, Champaign, IL.

Kuhn, T. S. 1962. *The structure of scientific revolutions*, Chicago, Chicago University Press.

Kutchins, H. & Kirk, S. 1997. *Making us crazy: DSM: The psychiatric bible and the creation of mental illness*, New York, The Free Press.

Lynch, T. 2001. *Beyond Prozac: Healing mental suffering without drugs*, Dublin, Mercier Press.

MacGabhann, L. 2014. Medicalisation and professionalization of mental health service delivery. *In:* Higgins, A. & McDaid, S. (eds.) *Mental health in Ireland: Policy, practice and law* (pp. 24–42), Dublin, Gill & Macmillan.

Maudsley, H. 1895. *The pathology of mind*, London, Julian Friedman Publishers.

McDaid, S. 2014. Shadow lives: Social exclusion and discrimination in the mental health context. *In*: Higgins, A. & McDaid, S. (eds.) *Mental health in Ireland: Policy, practice and law* (pp. 43–60), Dublin, Gill & Macmillan.

Moncrieff, J. 2007. *The myth of the chemical cure: A critique of psychiatric drug treatment*, London, Palgrave Macmillan.

Mosher, L. & Menn, A. 1970. Community residential treatment for schizophrenia: Two-year follow-up. *Psychiatric Services*, 29, 715–723.

National Disability Authority 2011. *A national survey of public attitudes to disability in Ireland*, Dublin, National Disability Authority.

Nolan, P. 1993. *A history of mental health nursing*, London, Chapman and Hall.

Rappaport, J. 1998. The art of social change: Community narratives as resources for individual and collective identity. *In*: Arriaga, X. B. & Oskamp, S. (eds.) *Addressing community problems: Psychosocial research and intervention* (pp. 225–246), Thousand Oaks CA, Sage.

Rappaport, J. 2000. Community narratives: Tales of terror and joy. *American Journal of Community Psychiatry*, 28, 1–24.

Rappaport, J. 2005. Community psychology is (thank God) more than science. *American Journal of Community Psychology*, 35, 231–238.

Rosenhan, D. L. 1973. On being sane in insane places. *Science*, 179, 250–258.

Rössler, W. 2006. Psychiatric rehabilitation today: An overview. *World Psychiatry*, 5, 151–157.

Scull, A. T. 1979. *Museums of madness: The social organization of madness in nineteenth-century England*, New York, St. Martin's Press.

Shorter, E. 1997. *A history of psychiatry: From the era of the asylum to the age of Prozac*, New York, John Wiley & Sons.

Slade, M. 2009. *Personal recovery and mental illness: A guide for mental health professionals*, Cambridge, Cambridge University Press.

Smyth, M. 1938. Psychiatric history and development in California. *American Journal of Psychiatry*, 94, 1223–1236. Cited in Whitaker, R. 2002. *Mad in America; Bad science, bad medicine, and the enduring mistreatment of the mentally ill*. Cambridge, MA, Perseus Publishing.

Whitaker, R. 2002. *Mad in America: Bad science, bad medicine, and the enduring mistreatment of the mentally ill*, New York, Basic Books.

Whitaker, R. 2010. *Anatomy of an epidemic: Magic bullets, psychiatric drugs, and the astonishing rise of mental illness in America*, New York, Random House.

Willis, T. 1684. Cited in Whitaker, R. (2002). *Mad in America: Bad science, bad medicine and the enduring mistreatment of the mentally ill*, New York, Perseus.

World Health Organization 1979. *Schizophrenia: An international follow-up study*, New York, Wiley.

3 Towards recovery

Beyond the psychiatric system

When I was first diagnosed with a mental illness over two decades ago, the concept that I could recover and reclaim a life beyond illness was not something ever discussed by my treating team. In fact the opposite was discussed more vigorously: much time and effort was devoted to educating and convincing me that the illness was permanent, and most likely to prevent me from living a full life. Plans were drawn for my long term care and treatment in environments that risked disconnecting me from my roles, opportunities, rights and responsibilities. These are not the messages of encouragement and hope you would expect from professionals.

(Glover in Amering and Schmolke 2009:xi)

The 'contemporary recovery' story of mental distress is an emerging story within the Western world. It is a story, as Amering and Schmolke (2009:xi) suggest, that is illuminating some of the limitations of the prevailing medical story and one which commentators such as UK clinical psychologist Mike Slade et al. (2012) believe has 'come of age'. The concept of recovery is now acting as the guiding principle underpinning mental health policy in many Western and English-speaking countries, including Ireland (Department of Health and Children 2006), England (Department of Health UK 2001), Scotland (Scottish Government 2012), New Zealand (Mental Health Commission 1998) and the United States (President's New Freedom Commission on Mental Health 2003). It is also a story that has been endorsed by some members of professional groups within mental health, such as nursing (Barker 2001, 2003, Barker and Buchanan-Barker 2005), psychology (Davidson 2003, 2005), occupational therapy (Pettican and Bryant 2007) and psychiatry (Dogra and Karim 2005, Lester and Gask 2006, Amering and Schmolke 2009).

It could be said that the concept of recovery, defined as a return to the pre-morbid or pre-illness state, is not new. Indeed, within mental health it might be suggested that the idea of recovery has always been an aspiration of psychiatry, with 'clinical recovery' or the reduction, elimination or sustained remission of 'clinical symptoms' being the primary focus of pharmacological interventions and the biomedical model. Similarly, the focus on 'functional recovery' and maximising people's skills in order that they fulfil social and vocational-related roles has been the underpinning principle of rehabilitation models of care. However, within the more contemporary and emerging model of recovery, as it applies to mental health, the term 'recovery' extends beyond these professionally led understandings and objectifying discourses of psychiatry. Arising from within the service-user movement and narratives of people's recovery journeys through mental distress, contemporary recovery writings provide alternative understandings (Deegan 1992, 1996, 1998, Anthony 1993, 2000, Fisher 1994, 2008, Coleman 1999, May 2000, Ridgway 2001) by drawing distinctions between clinical, functional and personal recovery and between service-based recovery and user-based recovery (Slade *et al*. 2008). In addition to providing 'ecologically valid pointers to what recovery looks and feels like from the inside' (Slade 2010:2), personal narratives of recovery frequently provide oppositional perspectives on the biomedical narrative of illness and challenging perspectives to policy makers and service providers, the people who largely shape the psychiatric system.

Recovery: A personal process that belongs to the service user

Internationally, while there is an acknowledgement of the scarcity of research that explores recovery from the perspective of those experiencing mental distress and labelled 'mentally ill', what literature is available suggests that recovery is not something that professionals do to service users but rather a personal process that belongs to and is defined by the service user. In contrast to clinical recovery, personal recovery is spoken of as something very different to the absence of 'illness' or symptoms. Instead, emphasis is placed on processes of healing, discovery and rebuilding a worthwhile life. It also emphasises the centrality of reclaiming positive roles and self-identity, irrespective of whether the person continues to have distressing experiences or 'symptoms'.

Personal recovery is viewed as 'a deeply personal, unique process of changing one's attitudes, values, feelings, goals, skills and/or roles . . . a way of living a satisfying, hopeful and contributing life even with the limitations caused by illness' (Anthony 1993:17). Personal recovery is about 'a journey of discovery' in which the person develops 'personal resourcefulness . . . control, a positive sense of self . . . and rediscovers their voice and belief in their ability to live a meaningful life, despite the presence of challenges' (Higgins 2008:7). Personal recovery is also about finding meaning and purpose in life through engaging in social roles, relationships and connections or, in the words of Michael Ryan, service user and Advancing Recovery in Ireland National lead, recovery is about having 'someone to love, somewhere to live and something meaningful to do' (Ryan 2015). Recovery narratives also recognise that recovery is not linear but a complex spiral process of small goals and achievable steps, characterised by periods of growth, insight, achievements and setbacks (Leamy *et al*. 2011). The course of recovery is also understood as a highly unique or individual process, with no two people taking the same path or using the same benchmarks to measure progress or outcomes. In contrast to the passivity of the 'patient role', which is frequently the hallmark of the biomedical narrative, recovery is a very active process and requires the person to engage with and take responsibility for one's own recovery (Jacobson and Curtis 2000).

Davidson (2003:45), in a synthesis of autobiographical accounts of recovery and of qualitative research with service users, found several common themes running through people's narratives of recovery including:

> a redefinition of self, the importance of being supported by others, renewing a sense of hope and commitment, accepting illness, being involved in meaningful activities and expanded social roles, managing symptoms, resuming control over and responsibility for one's life, overcoming stigma and exercising one's citizenship.

Brown and Kandirikirira's (2007:7) work, commissioned on behalf of the Scottish Recovery Network, identified six internal and six external elements necessary to initiate and maintain recovery. Internal elements included:

- Belief in self and developing a positive identity;
- Knowing that recovery is possible;
- Having meaningful activities in life;
- Developing positive relationships with others and your environment;
- Understanding 'illness/distress', mental health and general well-being; and
- Actively engaging in strategies to stay well and manage setbacks.

External elements consisted of:

- Having friends and family who are supportive but do not undermine the person's self-determination;
- Being told recovery is possible;
- Having contributions recognised and valued;
- Having formal support that is responsive and reflective of changing needs;
- Living and working in a community where other people see beyond your 'illness' and
- Having life choices accepted and validated.

In Ireland, echoing much of the international literature, Kartalova-O'Doherty and Tedstone Doherty, in a study involving the recovery narratives of 32 participants who had used mental health services, noted that recovery involved processes of reconnecting with self, with others and with time. In this study hope, acceptance and validation by others, being listened to and an ongoing involvement in the community helped motivate a necessary decision to fight for recovery rather than surrender to the role of 'patient' (Kartalova-O'Doherty and Tedstone Doherty 2010).

More recently, Leamy *et al.* (2011) conducted a systematic review and narrative synthesis of the literature on personal recovery. Paralleling some of the ideas presented earlier, they identified five over-arching themes or processes that formed a recovery framework of connectedness, hope, identity, meaning to life and empowerment (summarised using the acronym CHIME). Connectedness emphasises the importance of relationships with, and support of family, friends, peers, professionals and the wider community. Hope, described as the 'emotional essence of recovery', refers to the centrality of people having a belief in themselves and a belief that they can and will overcome obstacles, as well as other people believing in their recovery potential. Identity focuses on the process of redefining and reconstructing a new positive sense of self through the learning of new perspectives about oneself, one's experience of mental distress and the world. As Young and Ensing point out, 'trauma leaves one not only with the daunting task of reconstructing a new sense of self, but also with the task of determining how that self fits into the external world' (Young and Ensing 1999:223). Meaning in life refers to the process of discovering purpose and direction in one's life. For some, meaning may arise from work or social relationships; for others, it may be derived from advocacy, political action or spiritual connections. Similarly, some may use traditional explanatory frameworks from medicine, psychology or sociology to explain and understand their distress, while others may use existential or other frameworks to give meaning to their experiences. Thus, as Anthony (1993) points out, recovery does not commit the service user to a particular social, psychological, spiritual or biological understanding of mental distress; instead, whatever understanding of their situation the person comes to is equally as important as the professional interpretation. There are many ways of understanding and responding to mental health problems, and as no one size fits all, it is important that all voices are heard in the development of a consensus on what facilitates recovery for each individual. Thus, the recovery approach requires that mental health practitioners not only use professional expertise as the lens of understanding but value the voice and expertise of the person.

Fisher (2008) argues that the way out for people experiencing mental distress lies within processes of empowerment, having a voice, self-determination and choice. Thus, the 'E' in CHIME stands for empowerment and emphasises the centrality of the person taking control and responsibility for his or her own life and recovering a sense of personal resourcefulness and agency. While people may take control and responsibility in a variety of ways, ultimately it is the feeling of control and responsibility that leads to increased confidence and trust in one's abilities and voice, which results in positive cycles of willingness to take on additional challenges and positive risks.

This narrative model of recovery is also described in the writings of Frank (1995, 2000, 2002) and can be discovered within the philosophy of Bakhtin (1973, 1981). Frank believes that illness, or trauma, has the power to create chaotic new stories which disrupt a person's ability to deal with life. In his view a person who experiences trauma is first of all plunged into chaos, a chaos created by the 'articulations of an inarticulate body' (Frank 1995:8). People emerge from that chaos through a series of quests, through the rebuilding of identity and through others actively bearing witness to their suffering. Slowly a new story is synthesised in which the meaning of pain becomes central.

Similarly, Bakhtin (1981) describes life as an ongoing process of re-authorisation of the self through inclusive dialogue and the appropriation of ideas contained in a heteroglossia of stories. While his ideas were not specific to recovery from 'mental illness', they include learning to deal with the alien voices of trauma and authority, and are therefore highly applicable to an understanding of recovery processes. Rappaport (2000) also suggests that recovery begins when individuals become involved in a potent community narrative that challenges and counters the dominant negative cultural and professional narratives in which they are immersed. According to Rappaport (2000) this healing community is not professionally led but involves the mutuality of equal relationships.

Recovering from what?

All recovery narratives and narrative studies, in different ways, reveal that people are not just recovering from the life circumstances or traumas that gave rise to their mental distress or 'mental illness' but are also recovering from the consequence of the loss of rights and voice that often ensue from being labelled 'mentally ill'. There is strong evidence that many people experiencing mental health problems and labelled 'mentally ill' do not have access to the normal experiences of citizenship and suffer social exclusion, discrimination and victimisation (Rappaport 2000, Goodman *et al.* 2001, Thornicroft 2006), as well as structural discrimination at the level of access to housing, education and employment (Morris 2005, National Disability Authority [NDA] 2006, 2011). MacGabhann *et al.*'s (2010) Irish study commissioned by Amnesty International reported 61% of their sample experienced discrimination by members of their families, 58% by mental health professionals, and 80% had been discriminated against in the area of keeping or finding employment. Public attitude surveys also suggest the presence of alarmingly negative attitudes toward employing people with mental health problems or believing that people experiencing mental health problems have the same rights as people without mental health issues to fulfilment through a sexual relationship, being a parent and having children (NDA 2006, 2011). Together these findings strongly indicate that the label of 'mental illness' carries with it many negative cultural stories which support Repper and Perkins's (2003) claim that recovering from the consequences of discrimination can often be more challenging than recovering from the initial trauma and difficulties. The internalisation of stigma arising from being labelled 'mentally ill' has the potential not only to undermine self-esteem, self-efficacy and self-confidence, but may result in the person withdrawing from social interaction and contact as a stigma-resistance or -reduction strategy. Thus, as Mancini (2007) and others suggest, at the heart of the recovery process is the transformation from an illness-dominated identity or 'master status' to one that encompasses personal agency and competence and a process of re-engagement and meaningful integration into community life.

In addition, a recurring theme within recovery stories is that people who have encountered the mental health services have to recover from the impact of coercive, oppressive and paternalistic practices, as well as the disempowering effects of the illness-based model of psychiatric care (Chamberlin 1978, Coleman 1999, Maddock and Maddock 2006). Experiences, such as being treated like a disease rather than a person, experiencing a lack of dignity and respect by professionals, having to endure the side effects of treatments and having to hand over control of one's life to service providers and accept the identity of a 'passive patient', all work against the will to recover (Kartalova-O'Doherty and Tedstone Doherty 2010, Kartalova-O'Doherty *et al.* 2012). Similarly, care that is focused on risk avoidance, medication compliance and symptom reduction seriously diminishes the autonomy, agency and power of the person (Ahern 2013). As Deegan pointed out nearly 20 years ago:

> In order to support the recovery process mental health professionals must not rob us of the opportunity to fail. Professionals must embrace the concept of the dignity of risk and the right to failure if they are to be supportive.
>
> (Deegan 1996:97)

An additional factor impacting people's recovery is to be found in the 'chronicity discourse' which pervades the narratives of some professionals. Communicating low expectations of a good future to people experiencing mental distress has been described as 'spirit breaking' and 'hope sapping' by service users (Deegan 1990, Slade 2009, Kartalova-O'Doherty *et al.* 2012, Higgins and McGowan 2014, Watts *et al.* 2014). It was this prognostic pessimism that led Ridgway (2001) to advocate for mental health to reach beyond the

> storehouse of writings that describe psychiatric disorder as a catastrophic life event and depict people who experience significant and prolonged psychiatric problems as progressively deteriorating, persistently impairing, and in need of life-long care; [and develop a more] enriching knowledge base and literature to guide innovation in policy and practice under a recovery paradigm.
>
> (Ridgway 2001:335)

Thus, for many people recovery is not just a journey of personal change or social re-connection with others as they overcome their experience of mental distress or 'illness' but also a process of recovering from the social, political, cultural and economic consequence of being labelled 'mentally ill', a process of recovering from the alien voices of stigma and discrimination that are alive within society and a process of recovering from the effects of disempowering and paternalistic practices and treatments within the psychiatric system.

Recovery: A transformational ideology for mental health services

While certain guiding principles are gaining consensus, such as the importance of providing a service founded on hope, connection and empowerment, the recovery story that is emerging from the experience of service users is one that embodies a transformational ideology marked by political and social justice goals. It is a narrative that shines a light on the urgent need to challenge the inequalities, injustice and oppression that prevent people labelled 'mentally ill' from leading socially integrated and inclusive lives through addressing the causes and consequences of stigma, discrimination and social and economic exclusion. Reflecting a different conception of mental distress and more in keeping with the social model of disability, within this view, society, as opposed to the person, is viewed as 'defective' and in need of an intervention.

Recovery is also a narrative that is endeavouring to transform the mental health services by calling for a fundamental shift in the way we think about and conceptualise mental distress. While the emerging recovery story respects and embraces the contribution of all theoretical perspectives, including social, psychological, biological and spiritual, it challenges both the privileging of one theoretical perspective as the primary explanation for and treatment of mental distress and also the privileging of biomedical understandings and professional interpretations over personal meaning (Higgins 2008). Within a recovery paradigm the person experiencing a mental health problem is the 'expert' in their own life and as such develops their own epistemology, explanatory framework or meaning, setting forth their own criteria for recovery and mapping their own recovery journey. Thus, mental health practitioners seeking to engage in recovery practices are challenged to rethink prescriptive practices and a 'one size fits all' approach. They are challenged to respect the uniqueness of each person's individual journey and 'truly engage in dialogue with service users and families so that understandings, solutions, and plans are co-constructed, and a "consensus reality" of what is "real" is continually produced' (Higgins and McGowan 2014:69). Practitioners are also challenged to recast their professional narrative to a more empowering, optimistic and hopeful narrative and recognise each person's capacity to recover and develop personal resourcefulness, whatever the diagnosis, 'symptoms' or problem. Another aspect of the emerging recovery narrative is people's rights to engage with therapeutic or positive risk taking, which may 'involve the person taking on new challenges leading to personal growth and development' (Slade 2009:177). Thus, there is also a call for practitioners to embrace the concept of dignity of risk and people's right to failure (Higgins *et al*. 2015).

In keeping with the belief that recovery from 'mental illness' or emotional distress belongs to the person and not the mental health services, the recovery movement also calls for a deep analysis of the way mental health services are organised and implemented, including a critique of how power is distributed and shared within services (Higgins and McGowan 2014). In doing so it challenges practitioners to work to actively redress the power imbalances that service users experience within services and move away from 'professional centric' services and embrace the concept of expertise by experience and the role of mutual help, peer support and peer workers (McDaid 2013).

Concluding comments

The recovery story is an emerging story within mental health. Like the medical or rehabilitation story, it is not without its critics and sceptics, and neither is it a unified story but a concept that has many meanings and interpretations. Depending on the focus of the teller, recovery is a story about the meaning of mental health that emanates from people's lived experiences of distress. In this context it is a story of hope, strength, resilience, opportunity and growth and one that encapsulates human connection, meaning and purpose in life. For others it has a socio-political and human rights focused story that calls for a challenge to the discrimination that is built into the social, political, and economic structures and systems that not only discriminate against people labelled 'mentally ill', but actively contribute to people's mental distress. For others, it is a story of opposition to, and a critique of, the current psychiatric system, including a critique of professional power, diagnostic labels and iatrogenic induced harm, as well as the type of evidence which underpins current practices. In this context it is a call for a radical transformation of how we conceptualise mental distress and how we respond to people experiencing distress, including a call to move beyond professional-centric psychiatric services and embrace less hierarchical models of support, for example, peer or mutual support.

References

Ahern, N. 2013. *A tale of two boys*, Boston, National Empowerment Center.

Amering, M. & Schmolke, M. 2009. *Recovery in mental health: Reshaping scientific and clinical responsibilities*, Oxford, Wiley Blackwell.

Anthony, W. A. 1993. Recovery from mental illness: The guiding vision of the mental health service system in the 1990s. *Psychosocial Rehabilitation Journal*, 16, 521–537.

Anthony, W. A. 2000. A recovery-oriented service system: Setting some system level standards. *Psychiatric Rehabilitation Journal*, 24, 159–168.

Bakhtin, M. 1973. *Problems of Dostoevsky's poetics*, Ann Arbor, MI, Ardis Publishing.

Bakhtin, M. 1981. *The dialogical imagination*, Austin, University of Texas Press.

Barker, P. 2001. The Tidal Model: Developing an empowering, person-centred approach to recovery within psychiatric and mental health nursing. *Journal of Psychiatric and Mental Health Nursing*, 8, 233–240.

Barker, P. 2003. The Tidal Model: Psychiatric colonization, recovery and the paradigm shift in mental health care. *International Journal of Mental Health Nursing*, 12, 96–102.

Barker, P. J. & Buchanan-Barker, P. 2005. *The Tidal Model: A guide for mental health professionals*, Hove, East Sussex, UK, Brunner-Routledge.

Brown, W. & Kandirikirira, N. 2007. *Recovering mental health in Scotland: Report on narrative investigation of mental health recovery*, Glasgow, Scotland, Scottish Recovery Network.

Chamberlin, J. 1978. *On our own: Patient-controlled alternatives to the mental health system*, New York, McGraw-Hill.

Coleman, R. 1999. *Recovery: An alien concept*, Gloucester, UK, Handsell Publishing.

Davidson, L. 2003. *Living outside mental illness: Qualitative studies of recovery in schizophrenia*, New York and London, New York University Press.

Davidson, L., O'Connell, M. J., Tondora, J., Lawless, M. & Evans, A. C. 2005. Recovery in serious mental illness: A new wine or just a new bottle? *Professional Psychology: Research and Practice*, 36, 480–487.

Deegan, P. E. 1990. Spirit breaking: When the helping professions hurt. *The Humanistic Psychologist*, 18, 301–313.

Deegan, P. E. 1992. The independent living movement and people with psychiatric disabilities: Taking back control over our own lives. *Psychosocial Rehabilitation Journal*, 15, 3–19.

Deegan, P. E. 1996. *Recovery as a journey of the heart*, Boston, National Empowerment Center.

Deegan, P. E. 1998. Recovery: The lived experience of rehabilitation. *Psychosocial Rehabilitation Journal*, 11, 11–19.

Department of Health 2001. *The journey to recovery: The government's vision for mental health care*, London, Department of Health.

Department of Health and Children 2006. *A vision for change: Report of the expert group on mental health policy*, Dublin, Stationery Office.

Dogra, N. & Karim, K. 2005. Diversity training for psychiatrists. *Advances in Psychiatric Treatment*, 11, 159–167.

Fisher, D. B. 1994. Health care reform based on an empowerment model of recovery by people with psychiatric disabilities. *Psychiatric Services*, 45, 913–915.

Fisher, D. B. 2008. *A new vision of recovery*, Boston, National Empowerment Center.

Frank, A. W. 1995. *The wounded storyteller: Body, illness, and ethics*, Chicago, University of Chicago Press.

Frank, A. W. 2000. The standpoint of storyteller. *Qualitative Health Research*, 10, 354–365.

Frank, A. W. 2002. Why study people's stories? The dialogical ethics of narrative analysis. *International Journal of Qualitative Methods*, 1(1): 109–117.

Glover, H. 2009. Forward. *In:* Amering, M. & Schmolke, M. (eds.), *Recovery in mental health: Reshaping scientific and clinical responsibilities* (pp. xi–xii), Oxford, Wiley-Blackwell.

Goodman, L. A., Salyers, M. P., Mueser, K. T., Rosenberg, S. D., Swartz, M., Essock, S. M., Osher, F. C., Butterfield, M. I. & Swanson, J. 2001. Recent victimization in women and men with severe mental illness: Prevalence and correlates. *Journal of Traumatic Stress*, 14, 615–632.

Higgins, A. 2008. *A recovery approach within the Irish mental health services: A framework for development*, Dublin, Ireland, Mental Health Commission.

Higgins, A. & McGowan, P. 2014. Recovery and the recovery ethos: Challenges and possibilities. *In*: Higgins, A. & McDaid, S. (eds) *Mental health in Ireland: Policy, practice and law* (pp. 61–78), Dublin, Gill & Macmillan.

Higgins, A., Morrissey, J., Doyle, L., Bailey, J. & Gill, A. 2015. *Best practice principles for risk assessment and safety planning for nurses working in mental health services*, Dublin, Health Service Executive.

Jacobson, N. & Curtis, L. 2000. Recovery as policy in mental health services: Strategies emerging from the states. *Psychiatric Rehabilitation Journal*, 23, 333–341.

Kartalova-O'Doherty, Y., Stevenson, C. & Higgins, A. 2012. Reconnecting with life: A grounded theory study of mental health recovery in Ireland. *Journal of Mental Health*, 21, 135–143.

Kartalova-O'Doherty, Y. & Tedstone Doherty, D. 2010. *Reconnecting with life: Personal experiences of recovering from mental health problems in Ireland*, Dublin, Health Research Board.

Leamy, M., Bird, V., Le Boutillier, C., Williams, J. & Slade, M. 2011. Conceptual framework for personal recovery in mental health: Systematic review and narrative synthesis. *The British Journal of Psychiatry*, 199, 445–452.

Lester, H. & Gask, L. 2006. Delivering medical care for patients with serious mental illness or promoting a collaborative model of recovery? *The British Journal of Psychiatry*, 188, 401–402.

MacGabhann, L., Lakeman, R., McGowen, P., Parkinson, M., Reddmond, M., Sibitz, I., Stevenson, C. & Walsh, J. 2010. *Hear my voice: The experience of discrimination of people with mental health problems in Ireland*, Dublin, Dublin City University.

Maddock, M. & Maddock, J. 2006. *Soul survivor: A personal encounter with psychiatry*, Sheffield, UK, Asylum Books.

Mancini, M. A. 2007. The role of self–efficacy in recovery from serious psychiatric disabilities: A qualitative study with fifteen psychiatric survivors. *Qualitative Social Work*, 6, 49–74.

May, R. 2000. *Routes to recovery from psychosis: The roots of a clinical psychologist.* Clinical Psychology Forum. Division of Clinical Psychology of the British, 6–10.

McDaid, S. 2013. *Recovery: What you should expect from a good quality mental health service*, Dublin, Mental Health Reform.

Mental Health Commission 1998. *Blueprint for mental health services in New Zealand*, Wellington, Mental Health Commission.

Morris, G. H. 2005. Pursuing justice for the mentally disabled. *San Diego Law Review*, 42, 757–778.

National Disability Authority 2006. *Public attitudes to disability in Ireland*, Dublin, National Disability Authority.

National Disability Authority 2011. *A national survey of public attitudes to disability in Ireland*, Dublin, National Disability Authority.

Pettican, A. & Bryant, W. 2007. Sustaining a focus on occupation in community mental health practice. *The British Journal of Occupational Therapy*, 70, 140–146.

President's New Freedom Commission on Mental Health 2003. *Achieving the promise: Transforming mental health care in America*, Rockville, MD, DHHS.

Rappaport, J. 2000. Community narratives: Tales of terror and joy. *American Journal of Community Psychiatry*, 28, 1–24.

Repper, J. & Perkins, R. 2003. *Social inclusion and recovery: A model for mental health practice*, London, Baillière Tindall.

Ridgway, P. 2001. Restorying psychiatric disability: Learning from first person recovery narratives. *Psychiatric Rehabilitation Journal*, 24, 335–343.

Ryan, M. 2015. *An experience of creating the partnership.* Advancing Recovery in Ireland National Conference, Dublin, Trinity College Dublin.

Scottish Government 2012. *Mental health strategy for Scotland 2012–2015*, Edinburgh, Scottish Government.

Slade, M. 2009. *Personal recovery and mental illness: A guide for mental health professionals*, Cambridge, UK, Cambridge University Press.

Slade, M. 2010. Mental illness and well-being: The central importance of positive psychology and recovery approaches. *BMC Health Services Research*, 10, 1–14.

Slade, M., Amering, M. & Oades, L. 2008. Recovery: An international perspective. *Epidemiologia e Psichiatria Sociale*, 17, 128–137.

Slade, M., Williams, J., Bird, V., Leamy, M. & Le Boutillier, C. 2012. Recovery grows up. *Journal of Mental Health*, 21, 99–103.

Thornicroft, G. 2006. *Discrimination against people with mental illness*, Oxford, UK, Oxford University Press.

Watts, M., Downes, C. & Higgins, A. 2014. *Building capacity in mental health services to support recovery: An exploration of stakeholder perspectives pre and post intervention*, Dublin, Trinity College Dublin.

Young, S. L. & Ensing, D. S. 1999. Exploring recovery from the perspective of people with psychiatric disabilities. *Psychiatric Rehabilitation Journal*, 22, 219–231.

4 Towards equality and reciprocity
Mutual help/mutual support

The most challenging decisions ahead are not how to increase access to professional services but how to maximise life chances and enable people with mental health conditions to make the most of their lives. The real challenge is how to do things differently and use resources differently: recognise the limitations of traditional professional expertise, the value of the expertise of lived experience and rekindle the belief that citizens hold most of the solutions to human problems.

(Perkins 2010:36)

At first glance the meaning of mutual support may seem self-evident, with little need to explore its meaning or origin within the context of mental health care and recovery. However, like all concepts, different terms are used within practice and literature; thus, some explanation is required. According to philosopher Arnold Patent, mutual support is 'a universal principle involved in all levels of successfully living together' (Patent 1995:5). Clarence Hamilton (2008) suggests that the sacred texts of most cultures contain a reference to the idea of mutual help. Common to Christianity, Judaism and Islam is the commandment to 'love your neighbour as yourself' (Isaiah 8:20). The ideal(s) of mutuality have also been at the centre of secular revolutions and communist philosophy which saw any form of inequality contained within traditional hierarchies as evidencing a deep-seated social evil (Marx and Engels 1848). Despite the value placed on mutual support by successive cultures, Perkins (2010:36) suggests its inclusion within mental health systems remains one of the biggest challenges in our professionally reliant society.

Biologists Humberto Maturana and Francisco Varela (1987) suggest that mutual support may operate at a much more basic level than the consciously social. All living cells use 'language' or communicate with one another. Communication is designed to bring about a constant state of healthy equilibrium through a self-regulating negative feedback loop, a process known as autopoiesis. Irish psychiatrist Ivor Browne (2008:246) identifies five different levels within which this principle operates: the cell, the individual creature, a collection of similar creatures, an aggregate of species and finally within the biosphere. The idea of the human being as an example of an autopoietic system(s) that is itself part of a wider system has implications for the structure of and practice within the mental health service. The current mental health system is constructed as a hierarchy rather than a network of essentially equal parts. This hierarchy tends to favour one view or monologue, the bio-medical model, and ignore or suppress alternative views as well as the views and experiences of service users and their family members, thus denying the possibility of dialogue and co-production of solutions. The idea of mutual support, which positions experiential knowledge and non-medical views as equally valuable, challenges this hierarchical organisation, which relies exclusively on a form of professional expertise (Watts 2014). The medically constructed model of 'mental illness' also views the human body as hierarchical, where the activity of one organ, the brain, unilaterally controls all the other parts of the physical system. Neuroscientist Candace Pert (1998) questions the assumption that control must necessarily be hierarchical, stating,

> A network is different from a hierarchical structure that has a ruling 'station' at the top and a descending series of positions that play increasingly subsidiary roles. In a network, theoretically you can enter at any nodal point and quickly get to any other point; all locations are equal as far as the potential to 'rule' or direct the flow of information.
>
> (Pert 1998:184)

In Pert's view, all parts of the system are equally important to the maintenance of that system, and so everything becomes relevant, with no one overriding locus of control. Each participating part is valued equally and the actions of each affect the well-being of the whole.

Mutual support: A non-hierarchical approach

Within the literature, terms such as 'self-help', 'self-help groups', 'peer-support groups', 'mutual help', 'mutual aid', 'mutual support', 'peer support' and 'social support' are used, with many of them used interchangeably. Katz and Bender created the following general definition of self-help which is still widely accepted:

> Self help groups are voluntary, small group structures for mutual aid and the accomplishment of a special purpose. They are usually formed by peers who come together for mutual assistance in satisfying a common need, overcoming a common handicap or life-disrupting problem and bringing about desired social and/or personal change. . . . Self help groups emphasise face to face social interactions and the assumption of personal responsibility by members. They often provide material assistance, as well as emotional support. They are frequently 'cause' oriented, and promulgate an ideology of values through which members may attain an enhanced sense of personal identity.
>
> (Katz and Bender 1976 cited in Katz 1981:135–136)

While Katz and Bender's definition is nearly 40 years old, it still serves to highlight the core principles underpinning mutual help or the work of mutual-help groups, namely the coming together of people facing similar difficulties within a non-hierarchical framework, one that emphasises equality and reciprocity. Indeed, Humphreys and Rappaport (1994) suggest that the term 'self-help', which is frequently used to describe mutual-support groups, is a misnomer as it does not adequately capture the mutual, egalitarian and communal aspect of the support element, instead, suggesting an 'ethos of rugged individualism' (Humphreys and Rappaport 1994:218).

Mutual-support groups also differ from the generic concept of support groups. While both support and mutual-support groups may include members who experience similar problems, in a support group, the group facilitator may be a professional, thus changing the nature of support from an egalitarian reciprocal process into a hierarchical one-way process. In contrast, within mutual-support groups, all people, including the facilitators, face 'similar difficulties' (Loat 2011:19). In addition, each member of the group is valued equally regardless of their level of education, with the guiding principle for decision making being one of shared values, with every member simultaneously being able to give and receive support (Watts 2014).

Emerick (1995) developed the following typology of mutual-support groups within the mental health field by differentiating them according to political ideology:

- Individual therapy groups, which focus on personal change or the individual.
- Social movement groups, which aim to reform the traditional mental health system.
- Combined groups, which aim for both social and personal change.

Mutual support: Benefits

The most frequently mentioned benefit of mutual support arises from the opportunity it presents for giving as well as receiving help. Riessman named this 'the helper principle' after he observed various self-help groups and concluded that 'the act of helping another helps the helper more than the person helped' (Riessman 1965:28). In Riessman's view, having the opportunity to help others instils a feeling of self-efficacy and competence. Riessman (1990), reflecting on the negative social and personal consequences of only receiving help, noted that receiving help tends to underline inadequacy in the one receiving it and to create dependent relationships. These relationships become increasingly unequal, increasing the social status of the professional help giver, who gains self-esteem through the act of giving help, a benefit denied to the person receiving help. He concluded that 'if help giving is so beneficial and help receiving so problematic, the task would seem to be to restructure that helping process so that more people could play the helping role' (Riessman 1990:31).

Mutual-help groups are often described as safe places where members find support and empathy and, through the sharing of their personal stories, find new meaning, understanding and identity (Salem *et al.* 1988, Rappaport 1998,

Hatzidimitriadou 2002). Borkman (1990:325) suggests that mutual-support groups can be thought of as experiential learning communities, where members exchange experiential knowledge with each other and provide opportunities for behavioural rehearsal and the development of coping skills around many practical aspects of living. In addition, research suggests that participation in mutual-help groups increases and promotes social networking, social participation and inclusion (Seebohm *et al.* 2013), an important dimension given the societal stigma and self-stigma associated with a label of 'mental illness'. Drawing on social comparison theory, Loat (2011) highlights the positive impact of lateral comparisons, as people's experiences become normalised when they meet others who are experiencing similar distress or share similar hopes, fears and concerns. The positive impact of 'upward comparisons' is also noted, as people compare themselves to someone further along the road of recovery, who then becomes a role model or source of inspiration.

In the context of the emerging recovery movement, social spaces, created through mutual-support groups, can also foster alternative conceptualisations of the meaning of recovery beyond the narrow clinical definition provided by the medical view (Davidson *et al.* 1999). In addition, people have the opportunity to become active participants in their own recovery and are free to use whatever framework they wish to make sense of their experience rather than being passive consumers of diagnostic frameworks, the received wisdom of the 'professional expert' and the technical approaches to care and treatment of the mental health system (Adame and Leitner 2008). McLean (1995) suggests that within mutual-support groups people are able to dialogically move out of the devalued and oppressed 'mental patient role', and, with others, they may find 'mutual validation of injustice [that] prove[s] a powerful antidote against feelings of incompetence and worthlessness, and their anger motivate[s] them to assume control over their own lives' (1995:1059).

GROW: An international mutual-help movement

This section of the chapter is focused on GROW, the mutual-support organisation that the participants attended. GROW is an international mutual-help movement working in the area of mental health, which began in Sydney, Australia, in April 1957[1] and rapidly spread to other countries, including Ireland in 1969. GROW was founded by a group of people who experienced serious forms of 'mental illness'. While not regarding themselves as alcoholics, they met through Alcoholics Anonymous (AA) because of the absence, at that time, of a mutual-support group for people experiencing mental distress.

The key person among the founding group was Con Keogh, a Catholic priest and theologian. Con had obtained doctorates in divinity and philosophy before experiencing a psychosis that resulted in his involuntary hospitalisation and receipt of diagnosis of paranoid schizophrenia. Perhaps what makes Con so crucial to GROW's formation was that he became the organisation's epistemologist, painstakingly abstracting common threads from people's experiences of recovery and weaving the evolving insights into a practical and coherent psychology of mental health that today underpins the GROW program.

In terms of Emerick's (1995) typology, GROW doesn't fit easily into any one category but combines elements of all three. GROW is primarily about self-activation and personal empowerment through mutual support but rejects the idea that mutual help is a form of therapy. Members are, however, encouraged to seek out different forms of professional help or therapy where such specialist help is thought to be of benefit. While GROW does not advocate on behalf of its members, part of GROW's program of recovery involves each person 'carrying the message' (of recovery) to others in similar circumstances (GROW 2001:5). GROW members therefore take part in educational programmes aimed at professionals and at bringing about change within the mental health system. Clarke (1992:8) notes that in an earlier classification of mutual-help groups, the GROW program consists of a written philosophy containing a number of principles[2] which explore the nature of mental health/distress, personal growth and recovery. The first principle, the principle of Personal Value, states,

> No matter how bad my mental, physical, social or spiritual condition, I am always a human person loved by God[3] and a connecting link between persons. I am still valuable, my life has a purpose and I have my unique place and my unique part in my Creator's own saving, healing and transforming work (humanity).[4]
>
> (GROW 2001:7)

This principle challenges the dominant cultural and historical notions that people with a diagnosis of 'mental illness' are social 'burdens' and are not entitled to full citizenship. GROW also challenges the notion that 'mental illness' is something that only happens to a minority, suggesting that the line between mental health and 'mental illness' is a line that passes 'down through the heart of every single one of us' (GROW 2001:42).

The program occasionally uses the term 'mental illness' (GROW 2001:42, 54) and views the nature of 'mental illness' and the process of recovery as complex. GROW identifies four factors that influence people's mental health: Nature (heredity or constitution), Nurture (society or culture), Personal Action and God (or overall cause; GROW 2001:44). While receiving a diagnosis of 'mental illness' can be the result of all these, including the abusive actions of others; in GROW's philosophy, it is the responsibility of the person directly affected to get well by challenging 'learned habits of false thinking and disorganised living' (GROW 1994:48).

GROW also acknowledges that diagnosis and professional treatment or interventions can have a place in people's recovery, as external forms of control, such as hospitalisation, medication and professional help, if underpinned by recovery values, may make the emotional chaos of 'mental illness' somewhat manageable. However, in GROW's view these should quickly lead to a process where external controls are progressively replaced by friendship networks, the development of a person's own resources and skills to deal with life. GROW recognises the spirituality of the human condition as central to recovery and describes two forms of spirituality: horizontal spirituality, which is present between people (love, encouragement or a warm smile), and vertical spirituality, which represents a person's beliefs and values (and the effect these have on thoughts and behaviours; GROW 2001:69). In keeping with the principle of mutual help, the primary helpers in recovery are seen as 'friendly human beings who know from experience' how to recover. 'All other helpers, including professionals, are necessarily subordinate, good in their place, but harmful when they do not make way for that vital self activation through mutual help' (GROW 1994:48). While GROW acknowledges the potential role of professionals and medication in a recovery process, the aim of professional help should always be to awaken a person's own resources for living. Similarly, while medication in times of severe emotional turmoil is viewed as 'a boon and a blessing' (GROW 1995:61), the long-term use of medication is considered undesirable and should 'be gradually reduced and finally terminated' (GROW 1995:63) when personal resources have been developed. In GROW's definition people are recovered when:

- They are coping well with their duties and feel basically secure and contented.
- They are friendly and co-operative with those around them.
- Their main habitual supports for facing life are built-in habits of personal maturity accompanied by an increasing awareness of the presence and power of a loving God.[5] Not the doctor, nor the pills, nor even the group.
- The old irrational feelings, which may return from time to time, don't change the person's thinking or behaviour.
- The person completely integrates their past 'mental illness' experience, that is to say, they don't fear relapsing, they no longer have any great sense of stigma, and they are even positively glad they had a breakdown because it turned out to be a breakthrough to better and happier living.
- They find an expanded mental outlook, where the quality of their friendships and their deepened spiritual life has made each one a new person.

(GROW 2001:41)

The GROW program only becomes meaningful through people's interactions within GROW events. Central to these events is the weekly meeting,[6] which is officially described as 'A school of living' (GROW undated:4). Rappaport (1988:4) described the weekly GROW meetings as 'the glue that holds a whole community together'. The aim of the meeting is to enable each person to develop their unique character and realise their own giftedness and value. Each person reveals him- or herself to the group by giving a 'personal testimony' or a weekly 'report on progress' and through their actions at the meeting. In this way, the meetings become places of reciprocal witness, a witness that at once acknowledges the suffering and limitations of each person but which also attests to the 'giftedness and potential' of each person (GROW undated:1).

As GROW is a mutual-help group, no one is present primarily to offer help to others, although each person is expected to progressively become more involved in both helping others and allowing others to offer help in return. Acts of helping and being helped become reciprocal bonds that animate the meetings. A second reciprocal bond within GROW is the activity of leadership. Leadership is seen as a shared responsibility and involves everyone 'to the extent that he becomes an active member, helping others as well as himself to find and stay on the GROW way' (GROW 2003:41). Leadership extends from leading the weekly meeting[7] to any positive or caring act performed within the group, such as making tea or just simply smiling at somebody (GROW undated:14). GROW members are encouraged to move systematically through three distinct phases of leadership in which they are known as beginning, progressing and seasoned Growers. A person becomes a seasoned Grower after a minimum of 3 years' membership and having fulfilled the role of group organiser or recorder, which are key to facilitating GROW's weekly meetings. Commenting on leadership within GROW, Zimmerman *et al.* (1991:7) noted a defining feature of GROW is that it tends to create 'undermanned settings', where new members are challenged to step forward to fulfil these roles, whether they feel ready or not.

The weekly meeting is only one small part of a much larger community. Members of GROW are also encouraged to meet informally in between meetings, and GROW holds regular socials, outings, training events, live-in weekends and workshops. Other activities, such as publicity and fundraising events, all provide opportunities for involvement in the wider community. Salem *et al.* (1988) noted that GROW was more than a mutual-help group, it was an ongoing community that

> extends beyond weekly meetings to form a community for living. GROW becomes an integral part of the individual's life. There is a strong emphasis on development of friendship networks and each person is expected to be both a helper and to receive help relying on the helper therapy principle.
>
> (Salem *et al.* 1988:407)

What does the international and Irish evidence say about GROW?

Research into GROW was initiated by its own leaders in the 1980s (Rappaport 1988, 1998, 2000, 2005, 2008), and since then a number of other studies have been completed, including one by the World Health Organisation (Turner-Crowson and Jablensky 1987), three in Illinois, United States (Kennedy 1995, Kloos 1999, Corrigan *et al.* 2002, 2005), four in Australia (Young and Williams 1987, 1989, Shannon and Morrison 1990, Kercheval 2005, Finn *et al.* 2007, 2009) and one in New Zealand (Clarke 1992). A number of smaller studies have been conducted in Ireland (Dunne and Fitzpatrick 1999, Dunne and Meehan 2003, Henry and Dunne 2003, O'Donnell *et al.* 2008).

Findings from these studies indicate that GROW supports a diverse range of adult men and women of all age groups, ranging from people living independently and employed to people with 'high levels of symptomatology who live in sheltered environments' and, most importantly, to a marginal group who may not be receiving adequate support from traditional mental health services (Salem 1987, Shannon and Morrison 1990, Henry and Dunne 2003, O'Donnell *et al.* 2008). Of those attending GROW in Ireland, 91% reported having received professional help, 85% had been on medication and almost 60% had experienced hospitalisation (Henry and Dunne 2003).

Some of the positive outcomes identified by previous research included clinical-focused recovery outcomes, such as a reduction in admission days to inpatient services (Kennedy 1995), a reduction in levels of prescribed medication and a reduction in reliance on professional services by those who attended GROW (Young and Williams 1987, 1989, Shannon and Morrison 1990, Finn *et al.* 2007, 2009). Based on a 4-year mixed-methods study, Rappaport *et al.* (1985 concluded that

> those in GROW for 9 months or more were significantly better off than those in GROW for 3 months or less, in terms of having larger social networks, a higher rate of current employment and lower levels of psychopathology on several dimensions including psychoticism and depression.
>
> (Rappaport *et al.* 1985:18)

Others report on more personal-focused recovery outcomes, including an increase in social and emotional engagement, self-esteem, the giving of help to others, a sense of community and friendship and a positive transformation of identity (Kennedy 1995, Corrigan *et al.* 2005, Kercheval 2005). Maton and Salem (1995) concluded from their work that organisations like GROW are able to facilitate transformation of identity by possessing the characteristics of an empowering community, which they identified as:

- A belief system that inspires growth;
- An opportunity role structure that is pervasive, highly accessible and multi-functional; and
- A support system that is encompassing, peer based and provides a sense of community and leadership that is inspiring, talented, shared and committed to both setting and members.

> (Maton and Salem 1995:631)

While many studies have indicated benefits of participation in mutual-help groups (Edmunson *et al.* 1982, Galanter 1988, Christensen and Jacobson 1994), a number of criticisms and reservations have been expressed. Mental health professionals often hold reservations about a possible clash between a mutual-help group's approach and professional mental health care models, fearing possible interference with clinical interventions and decisions (Henry and Dunne 2003). Some express concern that there is a potential for over-dominant people within groups to have a negative impact on other less articulate or assertive members and are sceptical that 'unqualified peers' would have anything positive to offer (Loat 2011).

Drawing on traditional research paradigms, others critique mutual help on the grounds that there is a lack of robust evidence to support claims of impact and outcomes, commenting that studies indicating positive outcomes are largely uncontrolled and non-randomised (Davidson *et al.* 1999), with a dearth of randomised trials comparing outcomes of support groups to treatments offered by mainstream mental health services. However, Finn *et al.* (2009) and others suggest that viewing mutual-support groups as alternatives to mainstream treatment is missing the point, as they are a completely different phenomenon, underpinned by different philosophies and aims. In their view, any attempt to either compare or randomly assign people to comparison groups is to jeopardise research validity, as the natural composition of the mutual-support group would be changed. There is no doubt that limited personal contact between members of these groups and professionals is hindering the development of cooperative relations and perpetuating professional centrism (Kurtz and Chambon 1987, Clarke 1992) and a belief that 'mental illness' can only be ameliorated through the highly technical procedures of professionals (Davidson *et al.* 1999, 2006) or a belief that mutual support is an 'optional add-on' as opposed to an integral part of mental health care.

Concluding comments

Mutual help, or what is commonly referred to as peer support, is another story that is emerging and searching for a voice both within and outside the mental health system. Although mental health policy internationally and within Ireland endorses models that embrace peer workers and mutual-support workers, professional centrism continues to prevail. Indeed, comparisons can be drawn between the hierarchy of psychiatric care, where one authority imposes a unilinear form of control on another, and mutual support, which argues that within a system all parts of the system are interdependent, equally valuable and relevant to the well-being and development of the whole system. While there is some evidence that suggests mutual-help groups, such as GROW, can enhance both personal- and clinical-focused recovery outcomes, few studies incorporated in-depth interviews with people who attend GROW (Kennedy 1995, Corrigan *et al.* 2005, Kercheval 2005, Finn *et al.* 2009); hence the need for a study that focused on people's recovery narratives and explored the 'active ingredients' within the mutual support process that enabled personal recovery.

Notes

1 The founding group chose the name Recovery to emphasise the goal and the solution rather than the problem (Keogh 1979:11). Recovery changed its name to GROW in 1972 to avoid confusion with the American organisation Recovery Incorporated.
2 GROW's written philosophy and principles are contained in a number of writings and published books: *Readings for Recovery* (Keogh 1979), *Readings for Mental Health* (GROW International 2001), *Growing to Maturity* (Waters 2005), *Collections of Personal testimonies e.g. Soul Survivors* Volumes One and Two (GROW in Ireland 1996, 2005), training manuals e.g. *GROW Program Training Manual* (undated), *GROW International Organisational Manual* (2005), *Personal Growth and Community Building through Leadership* Parts one and two (GROW in Ireland 2003, 2008).
3 Non-believers omit the word 'God'.

4 Non-believers refer to humanity rather than God.
5 There are many references to God in the GROW program, but alternative wording is provided for non-believers, and groups may, if they so wish, hold meetings for non-believers. New members who profess a difficulty with the idea of God are advised to substitute the word 'good' for the word 'God' to get an idea of its meaning.
6 Each member of GROW has an individual copy of GROW's program of 'growth to maturity' (GROW 2001) which they bring with them to the weekly meeting and which acts as a workbook in between meetings. GROW meetings have no dues or fees and are anonymous and strictly confidential. A GROW meeting takes place once a week and is limited to a minimum of 3 and a maximum of 15 members. A GROW meeting lasts for between 90 minutes and 2 hours. Members are expected to attend the same meeting each week, unlike AA, in which people may attend as many different meetings as they wish. The main purpose of the meeting is to help each person find a way towards recovery or greater personal growth based on their unique needs and situation.
7 New members of the group will be expected to take their turn at leading after a minimum of 3 months' attendance.

References

Adame, A. L. & Leitner, L. M. 2008. Breaking out of the mainstream: The evolution of peer support alternatives to the mental health system. *Ethical Human Psychology and Psychiatry*, 10, 146–162.

Borkman, T. 1990. Self-help groups at the turning point: Emerging egalitarian alliances with the formal health care system. *American Journal of Community Psychology*, 18, 321–332.

Browne, I. 2008. *Music and madness*, Cork, Ireland, Cork University Press.

Christensen, A. & Jacobson, N. S. 1994. Who (or what) can do psychotherapy: The status and challenge of nonprofessional therapies. *Psychological Science*, 5, 8–14.

Clarke, P. 1992. *Mutual-help groups and mental health professionals: Barriers and implications for co-operative relations*. Unpublished thesis, School of Psychology, University of Auckland, Auckland, New Zealand.

Corrigan, P. W., Calabrese, J. D., Diwan, S. E., Keogh, C. B., Keck, L. & Mussey, C. 2002. Some recovery processes in mutual-help groups for persons with mental illness. I: Qualitative analysis of program materials and testimonies. *Community Mental Health Journal*, 38, 287–301.

Corrigan, P. W., Slopen, N., Gracia, G., Phelan, S., Keogh, C. B. & Keck, L. 2005. Some recovery processes in mutual-help groups for persons with mental illness. II: Qualitative analysis of participant interviews. *Community Mental Health Journal*, 41, 721–735.

Davidson, L., Chinman, M., Kloos, B., Weingarten, R., Stayner, D. & Tebes, J. K. 1999. Peer support among individuals with severe mental illness: A review of the evidence. *Clinical Psychology: Science and Practice*, 6, 165–187.

Davidson, L., Chinman, M., Sells, D. & Rowe, M. 2006. Peer support among adults with serious mental illness: A report from the field. *Schizophrenia Bulletin*, 32, 443.

Dunne, E. A. & Fitzpatrick, A. 1999. The views of professionals on the role of self help groups in the mental health area. *Irish Journal of Psychological Medicine*, 16, 84–89.

Dunne, E. A. & Meehan, T. 2003. *Personal growth and community development through leadership: Evaluation of a training programme*, Kilkenny, Ireland, GROW.

Edmunson, E., Bedell, J., Archer, R. & Gordon, R. 1982. Integrating skill building and peer support in mental health treatment. *In*: Jeger, A. & Slotnick, R. (eds.) *Community mental health and behavioral-ecology: A handbook of theory* (pp. 127–139), New York, Springer.

Emerick, R. E. 1995. Clients as claims makers in the self-help movement: Individual and social change ideologies in former mental patient self-help newsletters. *Psychosocial Rehabilitation Journal*, 18, 17–35.

Finn, L. D., Bishop, B. J. & Sparrow, N. 2009. Capturing dynamic processes of change in GROW mutual help groups for mental health. *American Journal of Community Psychology*, 44, 302–315.

Finn, L. D., Sparrow, N. H. & Bishop, B. 2007. Mutual help groups: An important gateway to wellbeing and mental health. *Australian Health Review*, 31, 246–255.

Galanter, M. 1988. Zealous self-help groups as adjuncts to psychiatric treatment: A study of Recovery Inc. *American Journal of Psychiatry*, 145, 1248–1253.

GROW 1994. *GROW in Ireland: A celebration and a vision of innovations in community mental health*, Kilkenny Ireland, GROW.

GROW 1995. *Introduction to GROW: Enabling versus disabling help in the care of the mentally ill*, Sydney, GROW International.

GROW 2001. *Program of growth maturity*, Sydney, GROW International.

GROW 2003. *Personal growth and community building through leadership: Part one*, Kilkenny Ireland, GROW.

GROW Undated. *GROW program training manual*, Sydney, GROW Publications.

GROW in Ireland 1996. *Soul survivors volume I*, Kilkenny, Ireland, GROW in Ireland Ltd.

GROW in Ireland 2008. *Personal growth and community building through leadership: part two*, Kilkenny, Ireland, GROW. in Ireland Ltd.

Grow International 2005. *Grow International organisational manual – revolutionary transformation of mental health care through the provenly successful introduction of mutual help leadership among mental sufferers*, Sydney, Australia, GROW International.

Hamilton, C. 2008. *Buddhism*, St Petersburg, FL, Red and Black Publishers.

Hatzidimitriadou, E. 2002. Political ideology, helping mechanisms and empowerment of mental health self-help/mutual aid groups. *Journal of Community & Applied Social Psychology*, 12, 271–285.

Henry, J. & Dunne, E. A. 2003. *GROW Ireland questionnaire to members: Report of results*, Cork, Ireland, University College Cork.

Humphreys, K. & Rappaport, J. 1994. Researching self-help/mutual aid groups and organizations: Many roads, one journey. *Applied and Preventive Psychology*, 3, 217–231.

Katz, A. H. 1981. Self-help and mutual aid: An emerging social movement? *Annual Review of Sociology*, 7, 129–155.

Katz, A. H. & Bender, E. I. 1976. *The strength in us: Self-help groups in the modern world*, New York, New Viewpoints.

Kennedy, M. 1995. *Becoming a GROWER: Worldview transformation in committed members of a mental health mutual help group*. Unpublished doctoral dissertation, Department of Educational Psychology, University of Illinois, DAI.

Keogh, C. B. 1979. *Readings for recovery*, Marrickville, New South Wales, Southwood Press.

Kercheval, B. L. 2005. *Women's experiences at GROW: 'There's an opportunity there to grow way beyond what you thought you could . . .'*. Unpublished degree Master of Applied Psychology (Community) School of Psychology, Faculty of Arts Victoria University. Victoria, Australia. http://www.growinamerica.org/home/research.

Kloos, B. 1999. *Cultivating identity: Meaning making in the context of residential treatment settings for persons with histories of psychological disorders*. Unpublished doctoral dissertation, University of Illinois at Urbana, Champaign, IL.

Kurtz, L. F. & Chambon, A. 1987. Comparison of self-help groups for mental health. *Health and Social Work*, 12, 275–283.

Loat, M. 2011. *Mutual support and mental health: A route to recovery*, London, Jessica Kingsley Publishers.

Marx and Engels Selected Works, Vol. One. 1969. Translated: Samuel Moore in cooperation with Frederick Engels, Moscow, Progress Publishers.

Maton, K. I. & Salem, D. A. 1995. Organizational characteristics of empowering community settings: A multiple case study approach. *American Journal of Community Psychology*, 23, 631–656.

Maturana, H. R. & Varela, F. J. 1987. *The tree of knowledge: The biological roots of human understanding*, Boston, Shambhala Publications.

McLean, A. 1995. Empowerment and the psychiatric consumer/ex-patient movement in the United States: Contradictions, crisis and change. *Social Science & Medicine*, 40, 1053–1071.

O'Donnell, A., Watson, E., Morris, E. & Watts, M. 2008. *A survey of GROW membership in Ireland*, Kilkenny, Ireland, GROW.

Patent, A. M. 1995. *You can have it all: A simple guide to a joyful and abundant life*, New York, Pocket Books.

Perkins, R. 2010. Professionals from centre stage to the wings. *In*: Sainsbury Centre for Mental Health (ed) *Looking ahead: The next 25 years in mental health* (p. 34), London, Sainsbury Centre for Mental Health.

Pert, C. 1998. *Molecules of emotion: The science between mind-body medicine*, New York, Simon and Schuster.

Rappaport, J. 1988. *The evaluation of GROW in the USA and its significance for community and mental health*. GROW National Seminar, Sydney, Australia. Cited in Finn, L., Bishop, B. & Sparrow, N. 2007. *Australian Health Review*, 31(2), 246–255.

Rappaport, J. 1998. The art of social change: Community narratives as resources for individual and collective identity. *In*: Arriaga, X. B. & Oskamp, S. (eds.) *Addressing community problems: Psychosocial research and intervention* (pp. 225–246), Thousand Oaks, CA, Sage.

Rappaport, J. 2000. Community narratives: Tales of terror and joy. *American Journal of Community Psychiatry*, 28, 1–24.

Rappaport, J. 2005. Community psychology is (thank God) more than science. *American Journal of Community Psychology*, 35, 231–238.

Rappaport, J. 2008. Introduction of Kenneth I: Maton on his receipt of the 2006 SCRA award for distinguished contributions to theory and research. *American Journal of Community Psychology*, 41, 1–3.

Rappaport, J., Seidman, E., Toro, P. A., McFadden, L., Resichl, T. M., Roberts, L. J., Salem, D. A., Stein, C. C. & Zimmerman, M. A. 1985. Collaborative research with a mutual help organisation. *Social Policy*, 15, 12–24.

Riessman, F. 1965. The 'helper' therapy principle. *Social Work*, 10, 27–32.

Riessman, F. 1990. Restructuring help: A human services paradigm for the 1990s. *American Journal of Community Psychology*, 18, 221–230.

Salem, D. 1987. *The culture of mutual help: Characteristics of the GROW membership*. First Biennial Conference on Community Research and Action, Columbia. Cited in Young, 1991. *A Research Evaluation of GROW, a Mutual Help Mental Health Organisation*, PhD Thesis, University of Tasmania, Tasmania.

Salem, D. A., Seidman, E. & Rappaport, J. 1988. Community treatment of the mentally III: The promise of mutual-help organizations. *Social Work*, 33, 403–408.

Seebohm, P., Chaudhary, S., Boyce, M., Elkan, R., Avis, M. & Munn-Giddings, C. 2013. The contribution of self-help/mutual aid groups to mental well-being. *Health and Social Care in the Community*, 21, 391–401.

Shannon, P. J. & Morrison, D. L. 1990. Who goes to GROW? *Australian and New Zealand Journal of Psychiatry*, 24, 96–102.

Turner-Crowson, J. & Jablensky, A. 1987. *WHO survey on self help groups and mental disorder*, Geneva, World Health Organization.

Waters, A. 2005. *GROWing to maturity: A potpourri of readings for mental health (the "Lavender Book")*. Kilkenny, Ireland, GROW in Ireland Ltd.

Watts, M. 2014. Peer support and mutual help as a means to recovery. *In*: Higgins, A. & McDaid, S. (eds.) *Mental health in Ireland: Policy, practice and law* (pp. 99–114), Dublin, Gill & Macmillan.

Young, J. & Williams, C. L. 1987. A research evaluation of GROW, a mutual help community mental health organisation. *Community Health Studies*, 11, 38–42.

Young, J. & Williams, C. L. 1989. Group process and social climate of GROW, a community mental health organisation. *Australian and New Zealand Journal of Psychiatry*, 23, 117–123.

Zimmerman, M. A., Reischl, T. M., Seidman, E., Rappaport, J., Toro, P. A. & Salem, D. A. 1991. Expansion strategies of a mutual help organization. *American Journal of Community Psychology*, 19, 251–278.

5 Generating recovery narratives for this study

By telling stories to ourselves and others – in dreams, in diaries, in friendships, in marriages, in therapy sessions – we grow slowly not only to know who we are but also to become who we are. Such fundamental aspects of living as recognising self and other, connecting with traditions, finding meaning in events, celebrating relationships and maintaining contact with others are accomplished with the benefit of narrative.

(Charon 2006:vii)

The term 'narrative' is usually applied to stories borne out of experience and told by people who have not been formally schooled in any professional theory. Smith (1998:327) has described narratives as 'a basic and universal mode of human expression'. While Labov and Waletzky (1967:12) confine narrative to 'the oral versions of human experience', Barthes notes many different sites and forms where narrative can be found including:

myth, legend, fable, tale, novella, epic, history, tragedy drama, comedy, mime, painting . . . stained glass windows, cinema, comics, news item, conversation. Moreover, under this almost infinite diversity of forms, narrative is present in every age, in every place, in every society; it begins with the very history of mankind and there nowhere is nor has been a people without narrative . . . it is simply there like life itself.

(Barthes 1982:251)

In the chapter introduction, Charon (2006:vii) illustrates the importance that stories can play within the context of personal development and growth.

Narrative research

Narrative research is a 'common way of carrying out qualitative research, a method that has recently gained in popularity' as a valid source of knowledge (Holloway and Freshwater 2007:3). Although it exists in various forms and is one of a range of qualitative methods that include grounded theory, ethnography, phenomenology and case study, there is no consensus about the nature of narrative research (Creswell 2005). In its simplest form, narrative research could be said to be no more than the gathering and analysis of 'related' or 'told' personal stories about human experience. Holloway and Freshwater (2007) give the root of 'narrative' as the Latin *gnarus*, meaning 'knowing', while 'story' comes from the Greek and Latin 'historias', which also means knowledge (by inquiry). From these etymological roots, narrative inquiry might thus be defined as 'abstracting and separating individual experiences told as 'stories' from a web of cultural and professional scripts and conveying these to an audience in the hope of enriching understanding and identifying possible areas of constructive change (Holloway and Freshwater 2007:5).

Narrative research strives to understand the links between events and relationships experienced by the narrator and the perceived 'plot' or meaning constructed from those experiences.

Perhaps the most important feature of narrative research is that it introduces the idea that personal experience(s) of 'ordinary people' is a valid form of knowledge and has a vital place within the human sciences. Reason (2003:206) sees the science of personal experience as an attempt to move 'beyond grand narratives toward localised, practical knowings'. Hynes et al. (2012:163) views the use of stories as a form of 'epistemic participation (aimed at) the integration of different forms of knowing'. Indeed, the increasing popularity of narrative as a research method is said to stem from a disenchantment with traditionalist, positivist research approaches, which are seen as incompatible with the complexities of human life and human knowing (Gubrium and Holstein 2009). A narrative approach was selected for this study for two reasons. First, GROW members are familiar with the concept of personal narrative and storytelling and therefore should be at home within this type of inquiry. Second, Rappaport (1988, 1993, 1995) suggests that the process of recovery through GROW involves a narrative and identity transformation, arguing that stories not only exist, but they have powerful effects on human behaviour, 'as they tell us not only who we are but who we have been, and who we can become' (Rappaport 1995:796).

The study's aim and objectives

The aim of this study was to generate a second-order narrative that would enhance our understanding of recovery and recovery through mutual help. A second-order narrative is defined by Elliott (2005:10) as 'the account a researcher constructs to make sense of the social world and of other people's experiences'. A second-order narrative can serve as a means to the construction of a new theory or new knowledge and as such, may offer an opportunity to provide a counter story to the dominant biomedical and clinical recovery story of mental distress.

The objectives of the study were to:

- Explore the recovery stories of a number of GROW leaders;
- Elucidate their collective recovery experiences; and
- Describe how various types of help facilitated, aided or impeded recovery.

The study location and participants

The study was conducted among members of GROW in Ireland. To be involved, participants had to have a minimum of 3 years involvement in GROW, have been involved in GROW leadership[1] at a formal level, have received a diagnosis of 'mental illness', been prescribed medication or hospitalised and consider themselves as having recovered. People were recruited through GROW fieldworkers, who circulated information and posters about the study to potential participants.

Ethical approval and ethical process

Ethical approval to conduct the study was granted by an ethics committee at Trinity College, Dublin, Ireland. Potential participants received written and verbal information about the aim and purpose of the study, the method that would be used to collect data and the procedures that would be used to protect their identity. Before each interview started this information was reiterated verbally, and the voluntary nature of participation and the right to withdraw from the interview process at any time or to request the removal of some parts of the interview was stressed. Any misgivings or questions were openly discussed. Participants were asked to sign a consent form and agree to audio recording before the formal interview began. They also gave permission for their stories to be published.

The difficulty of presenting data contained in the recovery stories of people involved in GROW and rendering them completely unrecognisable is perhaps accentuated by the fact that GROW is a relatively small organisation and each person may have told their story in different settings. The likelihood of people being identifiable within the GROW community is high. Participants assured us that this was not a problem. However, in order to ensure the maximum level of both anonymity and confidentiality, all participants are given a pseudonym. All references to the names of anyone mentioned by them, or the names of places and institutions are also changed.

Who were the people involved?

In total 26 people participated, 14 women and 12 men. Their ages ranged from 30 to mid-70s, with the mean age being 45 years. The average length of time in GROW was 11.6 years, with a range between 1.5[2] and 30 years. All participants had received a diagnosis of some form of 'mental illness'. Indeed, 18 participants reported receiving multiple diagnoses, with the majority having received up to four diagnoses. Diagnoses included schizophrenia, paranoid schizophrenia, schizoaffective disorder, bipolar depression, depression, anxiety, panic disorder, autism, agoraphobia, generalised anxiety, anorexia nervosa, alcoholism, obsessive-compulsive disorder and personality disorder.

All participants had been prescribed medication for their 'mental illness' at some point in their lives, and 15 (58%) people had been hospitalised within a mental health facility at some stage for their distress (three people had been hospitalised between 6 and 10 times). The participants came from eight of GROW's nine geo-graphic regions in the island of Ireland.

The vast majority of the participants were experienced GROW leaders and very proficient at facilitating GROW meetings. While 22 had served as group organis-ers and 16 as group recorders, they had also served in many other leadership roles, supporting newly formed groups, introducing GROW to the general public, serv-ing on regional and national management teams, representing GROW on local and national media or being involved in the development and delivery of training programmes.

Data collection

Data for the study were gathered through the use of single, audio-recorded, in-depth, unstructured interviews. These days everyone is familiar with the concept of 'the interview'. We live in 'an interview society, in which interviews seem central to making sense of our lives' (Silverman 1997:248). While interviews have tradi-tionally been asymmetrical, controlled through the use of semi- or fully structured interviews or questionnaires, narrative interviews move towards a symmetry of power, involvement and co-creation and are located at the low end of a continuum of researcher control. Unlike traditional research methods, in narrative research, interviewers do not try to be independent, objective, neutral or distant onlookers exploring a reality 'out there'. Instead, they act as a 'good host', make the person feel valued and at ease (Kvale and Brinkmann 2009:17), share control of the cre-ation of a narrative with the participants, and 'engage their emotions . . . [and] are empathic and close to the narrators' (Holloway and Freshwater 2007:3).

There is a growing awareness that meaning is socially constructed and that the interview itself has an influence on the type of knowledge produced. It is not a simple question of one independent person asking another equally independent person to reveal what they know; it is more a question of multiple selves and mul-tiple experiences within both parties dialoguing with each other to reveal unique and transitory mimeses of experience which are acceptable to both. Interviewers are not there to try and prove or uncover an 'unchanging reality'; instead, they are there to create an unthreatening space which encourages open dialogue and honest reflection and to listen to another's experience and his or her personal construction of their social reality. Interviews are acknowledged as 'space' between individu-als, where those involved have the power to enable or denigrate, build or destroy, nurture or abuse, reflect on or react to, or draw out or impose. Mishler (1986) suggests that the aim of the interview should be to empower the person. Empower-ment comes about in a number of ways, which include challenging and countering the idea of the interviewer as expert and through abandoning any preoccupation about research objectives, preconceived attitudes and ideas. Hence, the research-ers endeavoured to enter the world of the participant, see the unique face and hear the individual voice of each person being interviewed. Narrative interviewing is both art and science, art in that it concerns a creative act (co-creating a story) and science in that it is methodical and systematic (Holloway and Freshwater 2007).

Within this study the interviews were as unstructured as possible, beginning with a general question inviting each person to 'tell the story of their recovery'. The first part of the narrative interview concentrated on encouraging spontaneous storytelling with minimum interruptions, while the later parts were more reflective, with the researcher asking for more information about specific parts of the story.

Despite the fact that all participants shared very deep and personal reflections on their lives and this did at times bring up strong and vivid emotions, they were happy to continue with the conversation. Frank (2000) argues that caring for a person involves a willingness to witness that person's suffering. Indeed, the acknowledgement of the distress and a willingness to support the person through that distress was experienced as an act of caring witness and appeared to be enough to carry participants through these emotional parts of the conversation. Participants seemed genuine in their appreciation of the opportunity to explore and talk about their experiences with an actively interested ear.

Data analysis: The paucity of the written word

Conveying to the reader how the stories were analysed is a real challenge for a variety of reasons. Words evolve from within a human being, an embodied 'phenomenon' which, among many other things, contains memory, imagination and emotion as well as meaning (Rappaport 2000). They also evolve in the context of relationship because words are always spoken to someone. While the written word used in this book can span dimensions of time and distance and give an 'idea' of meaning, it cannot accurately describe 'how things really were' at the exact moment of utterance. It is almost like being given the words to a song without the music. To bring that song alive a conductor or musician would need to know each note and the strength and tempo with which it should be played. Even then two conductors would no doubt elicit different versions of the intended script. For instance, in Tom's story, the statement 'relationships were not a very successful thing in the family background', when read, seems to become a rather flat and almost quantitative fact. However, if you were present when the words were spoken, you would hear how they were spoken and enter into Tom's living world as he allows himself to remember the past. Just as Tom gets to the word 'successful' his voice breaks into a soft, almost disbelieving chuckle. This laugh contains incredulity, exasperation and loss at the long list of separations he has just recounted; his grandparents separated, his parents separated and his aunt who lived with them separated. Within that chuckle there are touches of despair; you can almost see and feel the horror he experienced at home as he allows himself to witness just how 'different' and 'separated' his childhood had become. There is also spirit in his voice. The spirit of a man who was told he would never work, never learn to drive and probably never have any friends unless he decided to live permanently in a psychiatric hospital. The spirit of a man whose life had been weighed down by intolerable side effects of medication and the horror of self-harm. It also hints at resilience – it is a brave man who can laugh at his own misfortune. Maybe the chuckle also contains his thoughts about his own future. Who knows? Today, Tom is married, runs a successful business, is deeply involved in numerous community projects and is in love with gardening. He has not taken psychotropic medication for more than 20 years.

We tell you a little about Tom here so you get a sense that it is impossible to capture within the forthcoming pages the human richness of each person's many and individual experiences. We tell you also so you can appreciate that it is impossible to describe exactly how the analysis took place, bar to say that each interview was listened to on numerous occasions and effort was made to get inside the experience of each person, to search for commonality and points of difference and provide as rich a description as possible to the reader.

Analysis method: The procedure

Before a formal process of analysis took place each interview was carefully transcribed, cleared of any identifying information and given a pseudonym to protect the person's identity. Analysis began with an immersion and familiarisation of each story as a 'whole entity'. This was achieved by listening to the recording while reading the transcript and by making notes in the margin. A short synopsis of each narrative was made, noting down the main plots contained within each story. These synopses were then re-read to see what subplots they contained. As the stories were worked through it slowly became obvious that each story naturally fell into three separate sections. Each contained descriptions of what life was like before attending GROW, what happened to them within GROW and what happened to people as they expanded their lives to ever larger social involvements in the wider GROW community and then society. It was also apparent that each story contained descriptions of the onset of severe distress, a process of isolation in a somatic and emotional body which became 'a place of terror'. Each person described becoming trapped in this physical body that was dominated by negative, often reactive and destructive feelings, feelings that robbed them of their ability to think 'rationally' (although they retained their ability to think logically).

Equally powerful were the positive descriptions of feelings experienced on coming into contact with GROW. Without exception, people reported quite dramatic and instant changes in their feelings once they had become involved in GROW. These changes were sustained as they became more and more involved. GROW represented 'a time of healing', a period where others became a second kind of self. This healing period was not the end of the process of recovery, rather a preparation. As several people suggested, GROW acted as a connecting link between 'illness and life'. There came a point where people began to choose what kind of life they wished to live. They actively began to seek 'niches' in society where they could develop their personal 'goals', exercise their new found ability to choose and develop their own unique character. It was from this thinking that the analysis of each person's story evolved in a more in-depth and comprehensive manner, and culminated in a recovery process titled a 're-enchantment with life'. Re-enchantment took place in three distinct but nonlinear phases described as moving from 'a place of terror' to a 'a time of healing' and finally to a place conceptualised as 'an opportunity to become'. The first theme, 'a place of terror', describes and explores the experience of 'being' in isolation. The second theme, 'a time of healing', explores people's experience of GROW membership, and finally the last theme 'an opportunity to become', examines the delight at finding a meaningful life through a selective involvement in society.

Concluding comments

Narrative research is based on the lived experience of those taking part. One of its strengths as a methodology is its privileging of people's stories as a valid form of knowledge, thus challenging traditional understandings of research and knowledge production. As a research methodology it is well aligned with the narrative focus of GROW work and with the democratic principles underpinning the philosophy of recovery and mutual support. It is also sufficiently flexible to allow each person's uniqueness to emerge, giving primacy to the person's voice in the telling, while enabling a second-order narrative of recovery through mutual support to be constructed. In the next section of this book people's stories of recovery, experienced as a 're-enchantment with life', unfold using a combination of participants' own words and ours. However, in the spirit of narrative work and in an attempt not to colonise participants' life worlds with our interpretations, primacy is given to the words of the people who shared their stories with us.

Notes

1 Leadership in GROW is divided into three levels of involvement. In the first 6 months of membership 'beginning GROWers' learn to be involved in many shared acts of group leadership. After this period 'progressing GROWers' take on formal leadership roles within the group or within a GROW fieldworker unit. 'Seasoned Growers', which is the category of leadership from whom this sample has been drawn, will have had a minimum of 3 years' GROW membership and will be involved in GROW's management regionally or nationally.
2 While inclusion criteria stipulated a minimum of 3 years in GROW one person was accepted for the study who had only been involved for 18 months. As this only became apparent at the beginning of the interview and as there was a considerable distance involved in travel, she was included and her story was used to explore any potential differences when compared to others with a much longer involvement in GROW.

References

Barthes, R. 1982. *La Littérature et réalité*, Paris, Editions Du Seuil.
Charon, R. 2006. *Narrative medicine: Honoring the stories of illness*, Oxford, UK, Oxford University Press.
Creswell, J. 2005. *Research design: Qualitative, quantitative, and mixed methods approaches*, New Delhi, Sage.
Elliott, J. 2005. *Using narrative in social research: Qualitative and quantitative approaches*, Los Angeles, Sage.
Frank, A. W. 2000. The standpoint of storyteller. *Qualitative Health Research*, 10, 354–365.
Gubrium, J. F. & Holstein, J. A. 2009. *Analyzing narrative reality*, Los Angeles, Sage.

Holloway, I. & Freshwater, D. 2007. *Narrative research in nursing*, London, Blackwell Publishing.

Hynes, G., Coghlan, D. & McCarron, M. 2012. Developing practice in healthcare: The contribution of building to negotiating the tensions among practical, professional and organisational knowing. *International Journal of Action Research*, 8, 159–184.

Kvale, S. & Brinkmann, S. 2009. *Interviews: Learning the craft of qualitative research interviewing*, London, Sage.

Labov, W. & Waletzky, J. 1967. Narrative analysis: Oral versions of personal experience. *Journal of Narrative and Life History*, 7, 3–38.

Mishler, E. 1986. *Research interviewing: Context and narrative*, London, Harvard University Press.

Rappaport, J. 1988. *The evaluation of GROW in the USA and its significance for community and mental health*. GROW National Seminar, Sydney. Cited in Finn, L., Bishop, B. & Sparrow, N. 2007. *Australian Health Review*, 31(2), 246–255.

Rappaport, J. 1993. Narrative studies, personal stories, and identity transformation in the mutual help context. *The Journal of Applied Behavioral Science*, 29, 239–256.

Rappaport, J. 1995. Empowerment meets narrative: Listening to stories and creating settings. *American Journal of Community Psychology*, 23, 795–807.

Rappaport, J. 2000. Community narratives: Tales of terror and joy. *American Journal of Community Psychiatry*, 28, 1–24.

Reason, P. 2003. Pragmatist philosophy and action research readings and conversation with Richard Rorty. *Action Research*, 1, 103–123.

Silverman, H. J. 1997. *Inscriptions: After phenomenology and structuralism*, Evanston, IL, Northwestern University Press.

Smith, M. 1998. *Social science in question*, London, Sage Publications Ltd & The Open University.

6 Personal journeys into severe emotional distress

I was a very nervous child I suppose, very nervous and I felt very inadequate. It was like as if I expected something awful was going to happen to me all the time, that feeling of doom and gloom. I didn't feel the world was a safe place to be. And my needs weren't met really. My mother, God love her, she got the dinner on the table and that was as far as it went. I suppose, in a way I was a bit pre-destined to mental illness and nerves, as you'd call it then. Because subsequently I realized, when I was growing up, he [my father] suffered with his nerves, and I think he drank to basically help him cope with life.

(Nan)

While the main aim of the research was to explore processes involved in recovery from 'mental illness' or severe emotional distress through mutual help, sooner or later, in the course of the interviews, each and every person described events and relationships which precipitated feelings of overwhelming distress that cumulatively led to a medical diagnosis of 'mental illness'. Participants' narratives chronicled a progressive descent into and entrapment within what some described as 'a place of terror'.

Entering a place of terror

While the primary cause of 'terror' could be close to home and involve the behaviour of one or two specific individuals, most participants described multiple sources of emotional distress emanating from within many levels of their wide social network. Events and experiences involving family, school, peers, and 'authoritative' others provided a consistent stream of negative emotional feedback. Each person's story provided evidence of them being involved in many traumatic events, such as physical and sexual abuse, bullying, family dysfunction, neglect, poverty and tragedy.

Developmental psychologist Urie Bronfenbrenner (1977:513) uses the term 'proximal processes' to describe negative experiences 'that occur in the immediate settings containing the developing person, and the larger social contexts, both formal and informal in which these settings are embedded' (Bronfenbrenner 1977). Richard described many such processes that contributed to his emotional distress. Richard's testimony began with school, where he spoke of the impact of negative experiences within the school environment:

> I had learning difficulties as a kid, I couldn't please my teachers, attention deficit disorder (ADD) or something. I managed to come 33rd in a class of 33 several years in a row.
>
> (Richard)

With a diagnosis of attention deficit disorder (ADD), the medical view might explain Richard's situation as stemming from a neurological disturbance within his brain. However, his story soon revealed a multitude of other social and cultural contexts, all of which collectively contributed to his growing sense of terror and emotional distress. His family, his 'immediate setting', was strained to its limits.

> My mother was over in England, and for her it was really foreign. No family support, and the kids just kept coming, and a few miscarriages as well. She was constantly pregnant and having to deal with kids.
>
> (Richard)

Richard's primary source of nurture, his mother, was under immense pressure. Marooned in a 'foreign' place, with no family support, numerous pregnancies and the unrecognised agony of miscarriages, left her emotionally unavailable to Richard. In addition, Richard's father was also rendered inaccessible:

> My father did what was expected of fathers. Work all the hours God sent. He was a builder's labourer. Sometimes I wouldn't see him for weeks. He would be tired and wouldn't want to deal with noisy kids. Anything to do with children was women's work.
>
> (Richard)

Within this context, consistently negative messages from school and home, including physical abuse, led Richard to see himself as a 'bad person'. Richard's view of being 'bad' was further reinforced by a priest and, through him, by the supreme authority of God:

> I couldn't please my teachers, I couldn't please my parents. I came to think I was a bad person', and then. . . . 'What really put the tin hat on it, this priest came in to prepare for confession. And oh, he went into great detail about how awful we were. God was hanging on the cross because of my sins, and the only way to get your sins forgiven was to go to confession. And not only that, you had to be truly sorry for the sins that you'd committed, and what did that mean? It meant that you'd never ever do that sin again. You know, I was only eight or nine [years old], but I knew at that stage I had done things, and I'd said to me parents 'I'm sorry I won't do that again' and invariably I did. So I knew.
>
> (Richard)

Richard 'knew', at the tender age of 8 years old, that he was 'done for'. His mother, father, teachers, priest and now God were telling him the same negative story. He had no one to go to for reassurance. And when the family moved back to Ireland, where his father and, shortly afterwards, a best friend, died, Richard's life became a theatre of terrifying distress.

Pat described a similar gradual buildup of terror and distress implicating many of the same sources and introducing still more. Pat was the only child of a couple who married late in life and who tended to avoid social contact with other families. From an early age he had a sense that he did not fit in and, despite being close to his parents, felt he could never discuss the difficulties he had socialising and mixing with others. For Pat, a major source of distress was bullying by his fellow pupils and some teachers. Bullying was not only physical but included taunts that he was 'mentally ill'. He lived near a large psychiatric hospital and had, from an early age, absorbed negative cultural stories of madness. He found the insinuation that he was mad terrifying:

> I didn't like school. I was always anxious and nervous as a child. I was bullied. . . . Part of the bullying involved young fellows jeering at you, because you lived near 'the mental'. One time a [Christian] Brother asked me my address, and he said 'go and behave or we will send you into (name of hospital)' and the titter from the boys. I was humiliated . . . I never spoke about it at home.
>
> (Pat)

Charlie's terror was rooted in early family experiences and was precipitated by what he described as 'abandonment and physical abuse'. Charlie grew up in a family where he could find no one to take care of him. At the age of 11 he moved in with a neighbour who subsequently used alcohol and drugs as a means of abuse.

> I would have experienced abandonment from my mother at 11. I just craved her love. I never got it. I got beatings. My father would also beat me and as I was the youngest, my older brother would beat me too. I was very very young. I had no safety . . . I was 11 and the woman of this house was, I thought, offering what I couldn't get in my own home which was acceptance and love. But basically she was supplying me with drinks [alcohol] and drugs and there was sexual abuse.
>
> (Charlie)

For Vicky, the actions of a trusted and respected family friend who sexually abused her as a child became her primary source of terror and emotional trauma. Vicky's life was reasonably happy until this happened. When it did she found it impossible to tell her parents or any other responsible adult, which meant that the abuse continued for a number of years.

> He [family friend] used to come into our house regularly, you know. Because he was an older man he was respected and welcomed always. I was only eight

at the time and it [sexual abuse] went on for 2 years. It made me feel dreadful. Dreadful. I felt incredibly fearful but I, I suppose I knew there was something wrong, I knew it was wrong, but I didn't feel able to do anything about it . . . I don't know how I'd describe it. I just knew it wasn't right, because I knew if it was right, you know, why was he always trying to get me on my own, and why was I never supposed to say it to anybody and stuff like that. As an 8-year-old, how do you reason things out like that? And I think it did affect the way I was in later years because, I was a bit of a rebel as I went into my teens and I think looking back I think I was sort of fighting against everything, lashing out in a sense, you know. He [the abuser] is dead, but whenever I pass the house it gives me the creeps. It affected the way I was in later years.

(Vicky)

A significant number of the participants (*n* = 7) in the study, like Vicky and Charlie, reported experiences of childhood sexual abuse. Many research studies have linked the experience of childhood abuse (physical, emotional and sexual) to a range of issues in later life, such as behaviour problems, post-traumatic stress, relationship problems, low self-esteem and voice hearing (Kendall-Tackett *et al.* 1993, Weiss *et al.* 1999, Coleman 2004, Spataro *et al.* 2004, Romme 2007).

For others unbearable levels of emotional distress were triggered by unexpected life events. For example, Claire's son and grandson both died by suicide. Claire had reared a family in a small town, coping well with all the ups and downs of family life. Her son appeared to be a happy and successful young man who had a career and a positive future to look forward to. She was close to him and to her grandson, who were good friends. When the tragedy happened Claire was so shocked and grief stricken that she was 'hospitalised with a suspected heart attack'.

Sociologist Arthur Frank (1995) suggests that major life traumas such as sudden bereavement or the diagnosis of a terminal illness can often only express themselves through the physical body, in a language that is both articulate and yet 'beyond words'. Claire's heart, her love for her son and grandson, had been attacked, and the pain was first expressed through her physical body. It took time for all concerned to see that it was overwhelming 'grief' as opposed to a physical blockage in an artery.

Ruth, on the other hand, identified a life of gruelling poverty and hard work as her main source of distress. Ruth had a large number of children, experienced ill health herself and was bereaved by the death of her husband and mother. In addition, she had to run the family business to provide financially for her family. In an attempt to cope, Ruth, in her own words, 'put her emotions down', with the result that despite feeling intense emotions, such as sadness or anger, she could not express them.

You didn't have time. I've seen my mother, I've seen another friend and her husband had rheumatoid arthritis. She had fourteen children. And my mother says 'Mary how are you?' she says 'if I had time I would cry'. You see, the only way you could deal with life was to put their emotions down. I found that when you push emotion down, you don't express emotion, you can't express anger.

(Ruth)

Other people identified the use of a physical substance like alcohol or drugs as further sources of emotional turmoil. For example, Penny began to rely on alcohol when she became involved in a recreational club and was thrust into a leadership role within that environment. Initially a social drink helped her relax, but this soon led to an increasing dependency.

I became regional president in [names a year]. A lot of drink involved. I had to go around to all the regional things and present the prizes and things . . . there's a lot of drink involved, particularly everyone was buying me drinks so I kind of became dependent.

(Penny)

Similarly, James, a young man struggling to adjust to student life and social independence, reported that cannabis, which he initially found to be helpful, soon made his life intolerable.

At first cannabis was almost an escape. But then it started going the other way into a kind of bad situation. It was like getting on a roller coaster.

(James)

Living in the place of terror

Jerome Bruner, a learning theorist, describes encountering the unexpected as '*peripeteia*' (2002:5). He gives as an example the story of Little Red Riding Hood, who was greeted by a hungry wolf instead of the kindly grandmother she expected. A '*peripeteia*' is a turning point, something which dramatically disrupts the direction and expectations of a person's life. Charlie met abandonment instead of maternal love. Vicky encountered a paedophile in the guise of a trusted neighbour. Pat was humiliated by a teacher from whom he expected safety. In each situation, these unique traumas registered as terrifying sensations felt deeply within the physical body. They were somatic stories of alarm, signalling in the strongest terms that something was wrong, and a call for help and resolution. Sue reported that she was continually depressed as a child and would spend long periods crying. Her parents were constantly undermining her friendship with others, telling her that people 'always want something from you'. At the height of her difficulties, Sue became 'both agoraphobic and claustrophobic', being as she said 'afraid to go out and afraid to stay in'. She graphically describes how the terror experienced in her physical body gave rise to thoughts that in turn became a further source of terror:

I started having anxiety attacks, but I didn't know what was wrong like. And em . . . a lot of the time it would manifest itself as me being sick . . . Invariably wherever I'd go out I'd want to be sick . . . even like when we were going home and my boyfriend would be walking me home at night, I would actually be sick at the thought of going home. Physically sick . . . I don't know whether that was because my mother would be waiting inside the door with a sweeping brush or something (laughing), because I was out so late, or whether I was so scared that the relationship [with boyfriend] would end, but that's when the anxiety started. For a long, long time I was in and out of hospital getting physical tests done, you know tests to my stomach, tests for diabetes, tests for thyroid gland dysfunction. All those tests and nobody could find a reason.

(Sue)

A physical response to traumatic experiences also evoked chaotic emotions which, according to Arthur Frank (1995), disrupted people's familiar life roadmap and plunged each person into a growing sense of chaos. Overtime this sense of chaos began to give rise to an upsurge of powerful and valid feelings, each articulating very real distress. The following are indicative of what participants said:

It [sexual abuse] made me feel dreadful.

(Vicky)

It [sexual harassment by an employer] was disgusting, it was revolting, I was so distraught.

(Lynn)

I had this wild sense of upset and loss.

(Richard)

Participants aptly described how this distress began to undermine their ability to deal with life, creating a constant sense of unease, alienation and pessimism about the future, all of which cast doubt on their ability to cope.

It was as though I expected something awful to happen.

(Nan)

There was a lot of unease, feeling alienated.

(Mathew)

A feeling of not being able to go on.

(Danny)

Martin Seligman, a prominent American psychologist, has suggested that the experience of terror (phobias and panic attacks) sets in motion what he calls 'catastrophic thinking' (1995:63). In his view, the mind desperately seeks valid external reasons for feelings of terror. For example, a person who experiences a panic attack in a supermarket begins to associate supermarkets as being the cause of terror, when in fact the fear is probably related to some past issue, where a physiological response was initially entirely appropriate. In an attempt to find a reason, Charlie, like many others who had experienced abuse, began to blame himself when in reality others should have been held to account.

> You don't think of it as abuse. You internalise it and think it is your fault. You are kind of a lost child.
>
> (Charlie)

> I was sexually abused when I was young, it made it that I couldn't really trust people.
>
> (Danny)

Danny concluded that he could no longer trust any adult because of the damaging actions of one person, thereby ruling out being re-assured and listened to by a truly loving other. Both false conclusions set the seeds for an ongoing separation and alienation from others.

Over time, unresolved feelings began to affect participants' ability to deal with the world. Kate began to think that her death would benefit her family, and Nan began to believe that if she could hide from life the terror would go away.

> I had got to the stage where I felt that suicide was the only way out. Death became a better option than the pain I was in. I thought if I just kill myself, it will be all over. Of course I had a million excuses as to why and how my husband and my little girls would be better off without me.
>
> (Kate)

> My world just got smaller and smaller, the only place that I felt safe was in my bedroom . . . so I hid away.
>
> (Nan)

For all the participants, gradually everything became terrifying, they could no longer act 'normally' and they began to live in what Mikhail Bakhtin (1973) describes as adventure time. Adventure time represents a total loss of personal control. Things just happen, and life becomes uncontrollable. Tom described a terrifying personal crisis in which his own behaviour added to his state of terror. He used the analogy of shaking a fizzy bottle until it explodes to describe the growth of unresolved chaotic emotions, which erupted into destructive thoughts and voices, leading to an attack upon himself.

> The social problems I had, sort of escalated then. It's like a fizzy bottle, you shake it, its going to blow . . . my mind started really going weird and I started cutting myself, started hearing voices in my head. I was taking razor blades and cutting myself up, I belted my fist through a greenhouse, cut my whole arm deeply open.
>
> (Tom)

Mathew and James also described losing control of their thoughts and how disturbed thinking affected their behaviour, which in a cyclical process generated more feelings of distress and terror.

> I thought I had lost my soul, and the only way to get it back was to drown. I was very alienated and troubled.
>
> (Mathew)

> I was at my wits' end. My mind had lost the run of itself. I had no control over the thoughts coming into my mind. It was like driving a car with no steering wheel and no brakes it was terrifying. I was just sure there was a plot happening. It was a different dimension in terms of reality. I felt as though I had walked through a demented gate. At the height of it I was doing well to get an hour's sleep. I had very very vivid dreams and a lot of times I couldn't be sure if I had dreamt something or whether it was actually happening.
>
> (James)

Mathew and James both 'walked through a demented gate', entering a terrifying world where it was impossible for them to tell what was real or unreal. Unlike Tom and Kate, whose destructive behaviours were aimed at themselves, James sensed the problem came from others, and his actions were therefore directed at protecting himself.

> There was a lot of strange stuff going on. I started getting these waves of anger. I was in my bedsit alone and all these thoughts were coming. People were out to get me and I said well I'm going to go out and sort this out. I got a bread knife and put it in my sock. I went walking the streets. I thought everyone in the whole world was out to get me.
>
> (James)

Another effect of living with unresolved terror was that over time, terrifying feelings seemed to spawn other destructive emotions. A number of participants recounted the buildup of feelings of hatred, resentment, rage and powerlessness:

> I was so full of hatred.
>
> (Jess)

> I resented my parents.
>
> (Helen)

> I should have had rage printed across my forehead.
>
> (Charlie)

> Rejection that was a big, big thing.
>
> (Frances)

These narratives clearly illustrate the way violent emotions and terrifying thoughts escalated to create life-and-death issues. While a number of people reported suicidal thoughts and suicide attempts, and James had armed himself with a knife and could perhaps have hurt someone, each person still retained enough insight or control to stop themselves from taking their own life or actually harming others. However, for some the embodied terror did drive them beyond the limits of reason, with devastating consequences. For example, Paul began to weave the ordinary behaviour of others into a terrifying delusion and committed a serious crime while in this 'delusional state'.

> I was totally paranoid about my friend. I believed he was plotting to kill me. I had nothing to work against this idea. That was the whole centre of my belief . . .
>
> (Paul)

Paul's world had become a terrifying life-and-death nightmare. He had 'nothing to work against this idea' [that his friend was plotting to kill him], and there was no one he could trust enough to check whether his reality was true. Tragically Paul's body became a place of terror, where terrifying feelings spawned terrifying thoughts and terrifying thoughts gave rise to terrifying acts, and while in this state he killed his friend.

Arthur Frank (1995) identifies bearing witness to suffering as key to healing. According to Frank, unless suffering is witnessed by a sympathetic other, it remains as 'an embodied memory . . . a memory of experience now written into tissues' (Frank 1995:185). Indeed, a recurring feature within all of the stories heard was the absence of someone to tell. Vicky was unable to tell her parents about the sexual abuse by a neighbour, Pat felt he could not burden his parents with the abuse he experienced at school, both Charlie and Richard had nobody available that they could talk to, and Ruth said that even if she had tried to talk about her difficulties 'no one would have had the time to listen'.

The lack of a sympathetic witness was also a feature of Jess's decline into what later became labelled a 'mental illness'. Jess, a former soldier, recounts:

> I was in the army. A lot of negative things happened. Taking bodies out of the water that time the [names an air disaster]. You are overseas and you're looking at a fight. I was there when someone got shot. You never get counselling, just a pat on the back, nothing about the thoughts that are there in your head afterwards. Soldiers didn't talk between themselves, never asked how you felt. I was left with all this negative stuff.
>
> (Jess)

Jess also reveals a cultural story that soldiers [men] are not meant to be affected by [job-related] trauma, a belief that is in direct conflict with his own experience. Jess's suffering not only related to his experience in the army but included other forms of loss and grief:

> We lost 4 kids [children] through miscarriages. I just love kids. It all started to unravel and fall apart. Losing the kids was soul destroying, I often wished my life

was ended. I wasn't able to go to work. Just couldn't face being with people.
I struggled every day just to get out of bed.

(Jess)

The accumulation of unresolved traumas was in Jess's words 'soul destroying'.
The use of the word 'soul' hints at a different level of discourse and impact. Jess
is not just emotionally hurt, he is spiritually wounded. Unresolved emotional turmoil over time cut him off from any sense of hope or value and made it impossible for him to find any positive meaning in what had happened to him. Being
swamped by a toxic mixture of destructive feelings had the effect of shutting Jess
and others off from all the ingredients of mental health, such as feelings of love,
joy, purpose and value, thereby rendering positive feelings which feed the human
soul inaccessible.

Concluding comments

Participants' narratives contained many emotional descriptions of a wide range
of real and damaging life events that became 'sources of [ongoing] terror' and
contributed to each one being diagnosed with 'mental illness'. Terror was first of
all experienced as a somatic story, a valid physiological response to a traumatic
life event. It was a call for something to be done, a call for care.

While emotional distress could be experienced as the result of the actions of
others, through chance life circumstances or as a consequence of a person's own
behaviour, the fact that no one was there to listen, give witness or deal with the
resultant trauma meant that all the participants became progressively imprisoned
in a world dominated by terrifying and unruly negative emotions. An increasing
inability to trust self and others was central to an ongoing process of distress,
which began to cultivate harmful ways of thinking about and relating to self and
others. Life as a consequence became slowly transformed into a living nightmare
as distressing feelings fed off a mixture of other toxic feelings such as hatred and
despair. These feelings in turn began to negatively affect the participants' ability
to think rationally and behave in a healthy manner, which systematically shut
them off from positive relationships with others and exponentially re-inforced
terrifying emotional, cognitive and relational stories about life.

References

Bakhtin, M. 1973. *Problems of Dostoevsky's poetics*, Ann Arbor, MI, Ardis Publishing.
Bronfenbrenner, U. 1977. Toward an experimental ecology of human development. *Ameri-can Psychologist*, 32, 513–531.
Bruner, J. 2002. *Making stories: Law, literature, life*, Cambridge, MA, London, Harvard University Press.
Coleman, R. 2004. *Recovery: An alien concept*, Fife, IL, P&P Press.
Frank, A. 1995. *The wounded storyteller: Body, illness, and ethics*, Chicago, University of Chicago Press.

Kendall-Tackett, K. A., Williams, L. M. & Finkelhor, D. 1993. Impact of sexual abuse on children: A review and synthesis of recent empirical studies. *Psychological Bulletin*, 113(1), 164–180.

Romme, M. 2007. *Recovering from voices by changing your relationship with them.* Hearing Voices Congress, Copenhagen. http://www.voicesireland.com/marius-romme-recovery-from-hearing-voices/

Seligman, M. E. 1995. The effectiveness of psychotherapy. *American Psychologist*, 50, 965–974.

Spataro, J., Mullen, P. E., Burgess, P. M., Wells, D. L. & Moss, S. A. 2004. Impact of child sexual abuse on mental health: Prospective study in males and females. *The British Journal of Psychiatry*, 184, 416–421.

Weiss, E. L., Longhurst, J. G. & Mazure, C. M. 1999. Childhood sexual abuse as a risk factor for depression in women: Psychosocial and neurobiological correlates. *American Journal of Psychiatry*, 156, 816–828.

7 Attempting to escape from distress and terror

> So there was a lot of strange stuff going on in my thought process, then it started to turn a bit darker. And going from where I felt vulnerable and people were out to get me, I started getting these waves of anger. And [decided] I'm going to do something about this.
>
> (James)

Each person's narrative provided valuable insights into the dialogical processes involved in the journey into a place of severe emotional distress or 'terror'. The narratives illustrated how trauma evoked a strong physical reaction, which over time gave rise to feelings of terror, revulsion and despair. Destructive emotions undermined people's ability to think rationally and adversely affected their behaviour and relationships with other people, which in turn led to more intense levels of personal distress, isolation and alienation. As part of their recovery story each participant went on to describe various attempts to escape from their distress and reported that often these initial efforts only served to exacerbate their situation, as the care and witness they needed was not always present.

Attempting to escape distress

In an attempt to contain escalating levels of distress, a frequently reported initial strategy was withdrawal from all social contact, a situation which inexorably led to serious isolation and even deeper levels of alienation. For Peter, negative experiences, such as being taunted about his looks, being punished by teachers and being neglected by his family, appeared to justify a withdrawal from people.

> I experienced other people as being negative. I had no friends, not even family members. I became a very angry person ranting about the state of things. I thought what's the point of getting involved? People are just selfish.
>
> (Peter)

Kate similarly described withdrawal from social interaction because she felt nobody understood her:

I felt that absolutely no-one understood me. I felt that I was different. I retreated into myself.

(Kate)

Gretta, like some others, described deciding to give up work, thereby making the situation worse.

I got to the stage when I didn't want to go to work and I loved going to work . . . I was even worse off then I missed the company.

(Gretta)

According to Bakhtin (1973) an ongoing integrative dialogue with others is the process by which all of us maintain our sense of identity and value. Other people provide us with a sense of who we are and whether our behaviour is acceptable or not. Consequently, this withdrawal and the resultant absence of friendly feedback from others left participants, like Peter, vulnerable to waves of disturbing feelings that turned the dislike of others into a hatred of himself.

Mood swings. Self-hatred and dual personality. Mr. High, Mr. Low. Emotions all over the place.

(Peter)

While Peter and Kate described choosing isolation, other participants reported becoming isolated as a result of the actions of others or life circumstances. For example, some participants described having parents who discouraged them from mixing with others while others reported moving to new places where they knew no one.

A small number of people reported making radical choices that they hoped would alleviate their growing sense of distress, but in reality these actions only served to increase distress levels within their lives. Charlie's attempt to escape his own abusive family by moving in with a 'kind motherly figure' only placed him in even greater danger, as he said,

I went looking for safety and love . . . but it came at a [terrible price].

(Charlie)

Vicky decided to find employment to escape the controlling behaviour of her husband, which he expressly forbade her to do. When she protested he became sexually violent, undermining her determination to escape from isolation:

I wanted to take up a part-time job, he wouldn't allow it. We got into an argument about it. I was sick to my stomach at the thought of going [to work], because of the way he was. He was determined I wasn't going and to make his point, he, he forced sex on me which I now recognise as rape. I hated him for it, I hated him for it at the time because I felt so horrible and I felt so dirty.

(Vicky)

Vicky's and Charlie's descriptions of the impact of their attempts to escape from terror resonate with Martin Seligman's (1972) theory of learned helplessness. Their legitimate efforts to escape terrifying situations led to punishments which gave rise to feelings of confusion, anger and helplessness. Charlie blamed himself for being sexually abused by an adult and later became dependent on alcohol and prescribed medication, dependencies he finally left behind with the help of addiction counsellors and GROW, while Vicky gave up trying to escape from her intolerable marriage and became resentfully submissive. It was only when her children grew up that Vicky managed to successfully leave this destructive marriage.

Mathew had been hospitalised more than 10 times and had received various diagnoses, including schizophrenia and schizo-affective disorder. He described how, once when he was in what he called 'a psychotic or a bizarre mental state', he came to the conclusion that he was such a bad person that he had lost his soul and the only way to retrieve it and to escape from this truly awful state was to drown himself. He tried to explain the thinking using the concept of living in a 'mythological land', a time where life was in a 'different dimension'. He was adamant that he had not been trying to kill himself when he was rescued in the heart of winter, naked, from a river by someone passing by but that he was only trying to escape from a soulless existence.

> I explain it like you're in a kind of mythical land. You're around everybody else in the same dimension but you're in a different dimension, and when somebody says something to you, you're talking from an everyday place, but you hear what they're saying in a mythical version. Just say for instance someone says ah 'the heavens is pouring down' and you think 'ah yes compassion falls from heaven and we all survive on the compassion of God'. You totally take up what's an everyday innocent remark and you give it this kind of a spiritual, mythical spin. And quite often you feel like you've lost your soul, you're on a quest to get your soul again or you're on a quest to save the world, it's all this kind of, this mythical stuff you know. It's in every one of us, but when you're unwell you're in this different dimension.
>
> (Mathew)

Similar negative outcomes were reported by Penny and James, who recounted misusing substances such as alcohol and cannabis in their initial attempt to soothe or escape from their uncomfortable feelings. However, it was not long before the substance use began contributing to even greater levels of distress, with Penny being admitted to a treatment centre and James's levels of anxiety and distress escalating:

> The cannabis it made the anxiety worse. Probably made me feel more self-conscious in an extreme way, and that self-consciousness not only went into feeling self-conscious in crowds but in terms of my thought process, it became paranoid thinking. I was sure there was a plot happening.
>
> (James)

Accessing professional help

At some point in their struggles each person in this study reported seeking professional help in an attempt to escape from their distress or 'place of terror'. While
some people reported aspects of accessing professional help as beneficial, for
many others their experience of mental health services only served to provide
new stories of distress, contributing further to a sense of helplessness and despair.

French philosopher Emanuel Levinas (1969) suggests that care of a human
being consists of two parts. While one part may involve making professional
interventions, such as diagnosis and treatment, by far the most important form of
care is centered on a compassionate understanding of the uniqueness, needs, value
and the suffering of the one to be cared for. Care means 'gazing into the face'
of the unknown other (Levinas 1969:110). It involves the emotions, and most
importantly it involves the expression of compassion. Some participants provided
descriptions of occasional relationships with mental health professionals which
contained elements of this kind of friendly mutuality and compassion. Mathew,
who found mental health professionals as a whole very impersonal, describes
some positive interactions with nurses:

> I remember when I was suicidal in [names hospital] a very kind nurse brought
> me into his office. Himself and another nurse were doing paperwork. They
> were talking to me and they had a kettle in there. They got me a cup of tea.
> I felt better after 10 minutes talking, it took me out of that place which was
> great you know.
>
> (Mathew)

In just 10 minutes the nurses' 'kindness' took Mathew out of that place of terror where he felt suicidal and out of control. Their relationship shifted from
being hierarchical to reciprocal, three people sharing a cup of tea. Tom, whose
overall experience of seeking professional help was negative, described a healing relationship with a social worker who befriended him while in hospital. He
immediately recognised in her a spirit of friendship. She asked Tom not about his
symptoms but about himself, his goals and dreams:

> She asked me a wee bit about myself. I told her I was trying to get the exams.
> When trust built up I went to her home. It turned out that her husband was a
> teacher in the same college [I was attending] and he gave me some private
> lessons free. . . . She also arranged, through my GP that I would see a psychol-
> ogist. She said there is a 6-month waiting list but I will try and speed it up.
>
> (Tom)

Claire described a close and significant relationship with her doctor. After the
trauma of the death of her son and grandson by suicide, she was offered an
appointment with a psychiatrist. In this account the doctor recognizes and
acknowledges Claire's suffering, and she in turn is able to experience him as

caring and compassionate. By bringing with him a box of tissues he signalled that it was okay for Claire to be distressed, and that he was not afraid of her revealing her suffering and pain:

> I saw him go with the box of tissues the first day I went, and I wondered why is this guy doing this, you know, of course he knew what he was dealing with, that I was going to cry as soon as I started to speak about it . . . As it turned out he's from the town and I actually knew his family and his brother had been one of my son's best friends so I was able to speak, you know. He really listened, he was very good and very helpful.
>
> (Claire)

However, the common experience of most people interacting with mental health professionals within the formal mental health services was far from therapeutic. There appeared to be a consistent lack of interest in people as unique individuals and a lack of curiosity about their stories of suffering. Speaking of their experience within the mental health system, time and time again, people commented on how health professionals failed to acknowledge their social context, and failed 'to bear witness to their suffering or value'. Thus, many found neither compassion nor practical help. Moreover, their experience of mental health services only served to provide new stories of distress. For example, Danny, whose experience of being sexually abused as a child had undermined his trust of all adults, found his first visit with a psychiatrist distinctly disturbing and unlikely to restore that trust:

> He wasn't looking at me while talking to me. He wasn't making any contact at all. I was wondering 'what's he rambling about'. When I look back on it like when he was talking, he was talking and writing and writing and asking me questions, and writing but he wasn't actually looking to my face.
>
> (Danny)

Even when participants did meet with friendly professionals, the medical lens through which professionals viewed their world only served to heighten participants' distress. For example, David became involved with a friendly doctor; however, the overall effect of these meetings was still a reminder that he was 'mentally ill', a diagnosis that rendered him terrifyingly impotent:

> He would ask me how are things and we would get on well. I kind of liked him to talk to, he's good fun. So I'd go and see him and I'd enjoy seeing him. But he just prescribed medicine and he would confirm to me that I was mentally ill.
>
> (David)

When Tom questioned why the medication failed to alleviate his suffering, the authoritative response from the medical professional fuelled his growing sense of terror. It was not just the doctor's words but the 'embodied subjectivity' (Burns 2006) of his gloominess and his low level of expectations that left Tom feeling that even when the current 'rough time' was over, there was very little that he could hope for:

> And he sort of looked very gloomily at me, and he said 'well now Tom, you're going through a rough time, very bad time' he says 'I'm surprised you're actually able to go home at all'. And he says: 'Well you'll be on medication for life. I don't think you'll ever hold down full-time work. Friendships will maybe be difficult but you'll make friendships within the hospital'. He said 'You'll never drive. Never drive. You'll never have a house of your own. Never have relationships' all those things. It was a total write-off. It was huge. I would have been nineteen.
>
> (Tom)

Peter's doctor conveyed the same disempowering medical story by appearing on television, a media outlet that amplified the authority of his view by casting him in the role of expert. The effect of this was to rob Peter of any hope for the future and to remind him of the doctor's lack of warmth towards him, who he described as 'a cold fish':

> My psychiatrist appeared on television. He was doing research that maintained that people like me with 'mental illness' have different brain structures. He was a cold fish. I thought at that time that I was permanently damaged and would be stuck in some kind of workshop for life.
>
> (Peter)

Mathew also suggested that the medical and diagnostic lens of illness rendered him and his life experiences irrelevant to his recovery:

> They are really only trying to find out your symptoms and they are worried about medication. Is he drugged too much or not enough?
>
> (Mathew)

Kate and others like Mathew and David identified two other factors which they believed undermined the possibility of being listened to, understood and realistically helped. The first was an inability on their own part to identify and articulate what was wrong and the second was a lack of time on the part of the professional:

> The GP has an average of five or six minutes to give to you and you know I had no words to describe how I was feeling.
>
> (Kate)

> I can nearly count the times on one hand where a nurse would actually talk to me . . . even for 3 or 4 minutes. It just didn't happen.
>
> (Mathew)

The longest conversation I had with any professional was 10 minutes in 20 years. Extraordinary isn't it?

(David)

The prescribing and taking of psychiatric medication lies at the heart of the medical story of 'mental illness' and mental health service provision (Lynch 2001, Whitaker 2010). Indeed, every person involved in the study reported being prescribed medication, with mixed outcomes. In terms of benefits some people spoke of medication taking 'the edge off things or taking the edge off pain' (Peg). James viewed medication as helping combat his obsessive and fearful thinking, thus allowing 'a breathing space' for reassuring feelings of appreciation to emerge:

On the second week I was put on an antidepressant. I didn't find any effect, but one day I was downtown and suddenly realised I had been able to day-dream, like normal people. The fears had gone away for a while. For five minutes I found myself appreciating the flowers, so the medication gave me a little breathing space.

(James)

Paul believed that by slowing him down, medication paved the way for him to begin to benefit from more personal forms of help, while Claire was enabled to sleep by taking medication:

Medication has been a factor in my being in recovery. The medication just slowed me down. It didn't bring my thinking back to normal. The delusions were still very heavy. The first signs of recovery were after about 3 months on medication.

(Paul)

Medication was helpful, yeah it was, especially to help me to sleep at night, that's the main thing, sleep.

(Claire)

From these various accounts it is clear that medication may play a role within some people's recovery process. Medication helped reduce levels of fear, slowed down mental processes and allowed sleep. In other words, medication temporarily altered the person's somatic state, reducing distressing thoughts and thus providing a starting point for change. However, for many, medication also brought further challenges and difficulties. Peter's experience of medication was traumatic, he experienced what he called a 'high' which he believed was caused by the prescription of an antidepressant.

I found it traumatic . . . I went on this massive high . . . It felt like my brain would blow up like a balloon and burst . . . I discovered afterwards that if you are manic and you're given an antidepressant there is the danger it will send you too high and that's what happened to me.

(Peter)

Pat and many others described side effects such as tremors, nausea and, in some cases, dependency.

They [the tablets] made me vomit. I would go out and my legs would turn to jelly. You would get mentally confused, your hands would be shaking, you would start coughing.

(Pat)

The tablets started me shaking and shaking and shaking.

(Ruth)

I took on the responsibility of giving up drink and switched to prescription drugs which I ended up abusing.

(Charlie)

It dawned on me that I needed more tablets to get the same kick. I often took more than 16.

(Kate)

Whilst many of the participants in this study (16 out of 26) successfully left medication behind, this journey was not always easy. Many people spoke of the terrifying withdrawal symptoms they experienced when they began to wean themselves off medication. The experiences associated with withdrawal were even more terrifying than the worst of Kate's mental distress:

I suffered the most intense withdrawal symptoms. Oh Jesus I mean what never happened to me in my worse day of being ill happened to me when I was coming off of the drugs, I saw things that weren't there, hallucinations. And that was absolutely terrifying.

(Kate)

Peter found it extremely hard to wean himself off medication, and during this intense period of struggle he received no encouragement or support from the professionals:

The interesting thing when I stopped taking any medications the doctor stopped seeing me . . . saying, 'if you won't take it [medication] there is no point seeing me'. I sense he was waiting for me to crack up.

(Peter)

Tom had a similar experience when he tried to come off medication:

> Oh there was times I found I nearly ended up back in the hospital again, it was very difficult to get off. But I did get to the stage where I only needed the anti-psychotic [medication] occasionally, not every day. My mind thinking was a lot clearer, I was getting a lot of these drugs out of my system . . . [and then I returned to the doctor] and he sort of looked at me over the glasses, and he says 'Lad you're having me on! You just can't do without them! And so he says 'well, there's no point in you coming in here then, so I'll discharge you . . . Aha, but he says, he smiles and says, 'I think you'll be back sooner rather than later'. But I wasn't back for another 9 years, when he retired.
>
> (Tom)

Fifteen of the 26 people interviewed had experienced hospitalisation within the formal mental health system. For many the hospital experience was extremely negative and non-therapeutic, only serving to generate numerous fears, including the fear of being forcefully medicated, being controlled, being kept there permanently and the fear of stigma and discrimination upon discharge. Penny, like many others, listed a litany of events, people and surroundings within the hospital setting which added to her sense of terror:

> It was horrible! The door locked and you were sleeping in a dormitory upstairs at night. I was frightened in it. The men's dormitory was there and the nurses' office was between and they used to go asleep. Sometimes at six o'clock in the morning this man would walk in and say the 'Our Father' [prayer] and I was terrified. The toilets were dirty and it's one thing I'm very particular about.
>
> (Penny)

Kate described the environment as boring and non-therapeutic.

> Absolutely nothing existed, I mean the unit [inpatient] I was in was built in a square, and most of us just strolled around the square all day.
>
> (Kate)

The commonest positive experience of this aspect of help was the idea of 'hospital as a place of sanctuary'. For James, the sanctuary was from his terrifying thoughts and the terror that he might harm himself or others.

> When the psychiatrist said to me look, I think you should spend some time in hospital I was absolutely delighted. I was at my wits end. I didn't know where to go. I was having plenty of suicidal thoughts as well [as thoughts of harming others], I really couldn't see a way out. Yeah, it was just what I needed to get away from it like.
>
> (James)

For some participants hospital was also a place to meet other people, with some reporting that contact with other service users was the most helpful aspect. For people such as Gretta, peer relationships became the most important part of her hospital experience.

> To me, depression was the same as any other sickness. If you fall and break your leg you go to hospital. If you're depressed you go to hospital. You come home and off you go again. I went into the hospital then and in there it showed me a complete different light, because in there I was seeing people, a lot of people the same as myself and I saw then how they were kind of coping with it, and I wasn't the only one as miserable and there was a reason for it. The doctor wasn't really that helpful no, I really think I had more support from the people [other service users] that was in the hospital.

(Gretta)

Some participants, like Kate and Penny, reported that while in hospital they were introduced to the idea of peer-support groups or heard about GROW, an introduction that marked a significant moment in their recovery journey.

Concluding comments

Descriptions of how people tried unsuccessfully to escape from unique 'places of terror' brings to an end the first part of the findings from this study. Attempts to escape from unbearable levels of personal distress included a withdrawal from relationships with others, seeking relief through non-prescriptive drugs or alcohol and eventually, in all cases, seeking professional support. While some aspects of professional support were helpful, in general, all efforts to escape from the terror and distress had negative consequences, merely adding a sense of helplessness to the cumulative effects of unresolved trauma and further undermining people's belief in their ability to recover. Another common theme to emerge from people's stories was the continued lack of sympathetic witness, someone to listen and provide understanding and active support. The mental health system, parents, teachers and other potentially caring adults all consistently failed to provide a compassionate and listening ear, which might help remove the source of terror and empower participants to deal with its malignant effects. It was only when each person decided to attend weekly mutual-support meetings and access the help of peers that people began to find a way out of their terror and distress and start a journey towards recovery and mental well-being.

References

Bakhtin, M. 1973. *Problems of Dostoevsky's poetics*, Ann Arbor, MI, Ardis Publishing.
Burns, M. L. 2006. Bodies that speak: Examining the dialogues in research interactions. *Qualitative Research in Psychology*, 3, 3–18.

Levinas, E. 1969. *Totality and infinity: An essay on exteriority*, Pittsburgh, PA, Duquesne University Press.

Lynch, T. 2001. *Beyond Prozac: Healing mental suffering without drugs*, Dublin, Mercier Press.

Seligman, M. E. 1972. Learned helplessness. *Annual Review of Medicine*, 23, 407–412.

Whitaker, R. 2010. *Anatomy of an epidemic: Magic bullets, psychiatric drugs, and the astonishing rise of mental illness in America*, New York, Random House.

8 A time of healing

Struggling through fear to encounter hope and trust

At the start I resisted. I had been out of work for up to 6 months, you know. I just struggled every day to wake up and to get out of bed and realise that I had a life. I wasn't able to go to work, just wasn't able, just couldn't face being with people. It was a major struggle coming to GROW. It wasn't my idea at all. I knew nothing about that kind of thing. I remember sitting, six months actually, I'd sit in my car and I would go home and my wife would say 'well how did you get on at the [GROW] meeting' and I'd say 'it was grand'. If she asked me anything about the meeting I'd say 'I can't tell you, it's confidential'. You know I was even in that much denial in myself that I sat for two hours [each week] in the bloody cold. And I sat outside the building, then I got so bloody cold I had to come in [laughs].

(Jess)

Participants described a number of failed strategies in their attempts to escape from unique 'places of terror'. Avoiding social contacts, the use of alcohol or illegal drugs and seeking professional help had all been to no avail in bringing relief. These attempts often served to exacerbate people's sense of alienation and hopelessness and, in many situations, added another layer of despair, helplessness and disempowerment to their distress. As the participants' narratives unfolded many went on to describe experiencing an intense personal struggle in their decision to attend the mutual support of GROW meetings.

Struggling with fear and struggling to attend

After years of choosing to isolate themselves from others and being frequently let down by people they might have expected to be trustworthy, it was difficult for participants to overcome high levels of fear and ignore their grave doubts about joining a group. As Jess described in the introduction of this chapter, it took him 6 months to pluck up the courage to enter his first GROW meeting, as he 'just couldn't face being with people'. Participants' accounts suggested that the decision to attend, though often motivated by a desire to escape intense emotional distress and, frequently, a disillusionment with professional forms of help, was accompanied by a deep mistrust of and discomfort around people and an intense fear of more rejection and disillusionment.

> I just found it extremely difficult to be with people, end of story, no matter who they were, whether they were my family, whether they were in the street. So I just found it difficult to think about a group.
>
> (Kate)

> I was terrified of my shadow, when I joined GROW. I couldn't talk to people, I was terrified, and I had to force myself to go, I was not very good at forcing myself to do things.
>
> (David)

Similarly, it took Mags a very long time to decide to attend. She described how she had attended one meeting of GROW early in her struggles and had left it for 'a number of years' before making a second visit. Just as Jess, in the introductory quote, reported 'being driven in by the cold', Mags's main motivator was a growing sense of desperation over 7 years, which had included efforts to die by suicide connected to relationship crises. She had become increasingly afraid of her suicidal feelings and was increasingly disillusioned with her encounters with professionals:

> I had tried everything and I knew what was ahead. It [her distress] had been going on now for nearly 7 years. I had felt suicidal over the breakup of the engagement, I had 2 attempts [to die by suicide], and then this last time I was in hospital and I thought 'right that GROW crowd, I'll give them another shot' because I knew what plan B was.
>
> (Mags)

Peter went along because his experiences of the mental health system had become part of his despair. Perhaps GROW may offer an alternative:

> There was an article about GROW in the local paper. I went along because perhaps GROW offered a way out.
>
> (Peter)

Lynn was disillusioned with the empty promises she received when she looked for help at work, and despite being terrified that someone within the group would recognize her or that her harasser might be within the group, she eventually plucked up the courage to attend:

> I felt very apprehensive at first, would I know anyone for instance or would anyone recognise me. And I was a nervous wreck because I was afraid that he [her harasser] might be there, because he'd be one of these to get out of the problem he would nearly go to places like that.
>
> (Lynn)

Kate and Danny both reported attending rather reluctantly because a relative brought them along. Helen had real doubts about GROW and had refused to attend while she was in hospital. It was only when she met a nurse in the local community mental health centre who enthusiastically recommended that she should attend that she became convinced that it might help her and was thus able to put her doubts to one side.

> So I wasn't positive about GROW, and I wouldn't go to it in the hospital, but when I came out I started attending the community mental health centre because a nurse told me I should attend.
>
> (Helen)

Encountering a warm, compassionate welcome

Despite having real doubts about attending GROW, once participants did attend, each person reported a number of positive experiences and feelings which proved to be the start of their recovery journey. Participants described strikingly powerful and instant effects of receiving a warm, compassionate welcome from the other members of GROW. Words such as 'safe', 'wonderful', 'enjoyable', 'mind-blowing' accompanied by accentuating adjectives such as 'so' or 'really' all described spontaneously awoken and exciting feelings or somatic stories which acted as positive 'peripeteia', instantly opening the door to new life possibilities. There was a tangible realization that something positive and promising was taking place, a stirring which held an authenticity that was absent from previous quests for help. The welcoming warmth of others reached into hidden places in each person's heart, stirring up the essences necessary for the beginning of a real recovery, essences such as hope, meaning and belonging. There was a real feeling of having discovered a place where they belonged and were welcome.

> From the minute I went in the door there was a feeling of warmth, a feeling of not being on your own any more. A feeling of there's more people [like me] who just didn't happen to make it [easily through life]. It was a warmth, it was a smile, just the feeling of being here.
>
> (Cathy)

> At the first meeting, there was about ten or eleven people there and I didn't know any of them but the first thing they done, . . . they made me welcome and offered me a cup of tea, thanked me for coming along to the meeting and I felt really comfortable then.
>
> (Danny)

> I said this is great, the one thing that stood out amongst everything else was how friendly they were.
>
> (Pat)

It was as though the group acted as a powerful human tranquilliser,[1] which dramatically calmed the wild horses of emotion and released dormant resources deep inside.

> Like there were all these smiling faces around the room and . . . and they [group members] made me feel very welcome and that fear I had sort of left me, you know, I felt at home very quickly.
>
> (Penny)

> I'll never forget [names a person] and the smile on her face, she was so friendly and welcoming, it was the very same, it was your best friend that you'd met after years. And we went in and we sat around, and of course we were all nervous and very unsure of ourselves, and she was so nice and so lovely we thought God, is she for real? After I came home and talked about it and sure I'd give it another try.
>
> (Gretta)

Many other people commented on the relief they experienced at discovering that other people had problems similar to their own, a power which broke the sense of being totally different and alone. It also came as a real revelation to know that people actually talked openly about their problems, which in turn instilled a strong feeling of connection with the people present:

> They [the other members of the group] were people, looking for the same, looking for answers like myself. I got a sense . . . somewhere in the back of my head I could identify and relate to what was going on. So from the get go, I'd say I connected and I had lost that sense of connection with people, even within my family.
>
> (Kate)

Arthur Frank (1995) suggests that suffering is a call for compassion and that the necessary basis for establishing a loving community is the compassionate acceptance of others. Nan alluded to the fact that, even at her first meeting, she was unconditionally accepted for who she was; there was no need to explain herself or begin to articulate her problems, as the group understood her suffering and empathised by offering her a silent, compassionate welcome. This feeling of being understood offered Nan the promise of recovery, lifting her spirits and changing her emotions from anxiety to wonder:

> At my first meeting, I was desperately nervous, falling off the chair with anxiety. I can honestly say that was the beginning of my recovery. It was so wonderful. I felt if I am going to get better this is the only place that can happen. I didn't talk much to people and I certainly didn't share my problems, you know the anxiety, depression and all that, so to meet these people that

seemed to understand me was amazing, absolutely amazing. And after a few weeks I did begin to tell my story.

(Nan)

Peter, a man who declared himself to be an 'atheist/pagan', experienced a spiritual power emanating from a group of people sharing their life problems. It was something he felt transcended the individual human being and was perhaps the defining feature of the loving community to which Frank (1995) referred.

> There is something mystical about a good GROW group. You reach each other at a level of deeper understanding, and just this sense of shared humanity. You get a sense there is a spiritual presence.

(Peter)

From these narratives of people's early encounters with mutual help, a picture emerges of an awakening sense of belonging and unconditional acceptance. Many participants suggested that all these positive feelings and experiences constituted the beginnings of an ability to trust others and an awakening of possibility for the future which included the emergence of a sense of hope. Mags, who had put off attending for years, was at the nadir of despair when she finally went along to GROW. At her first meeting she recalled hearing a young woman telling her story of recovery. This experience not only encouraged Mags, but it positively challenged her because this woman's recovery involved suffering which Mags thought was much worse than her own. Above all, hearing this young woman's story gave Mags hope:

> She [another GROW member] was looking a million dollars, fully recovered and so warm and friendly. I felt that night going home that I had been lifted slightly. I felt I'd got hope and hope had never occurred to me before. I just feel today you can't go into a supermarket and buy hope. I think that's the very first step, hoping that, you know I can get well and stay well. That was the start. The example of this other person in the group who made such a huge recovery from such unthinkable and terrifying stuff.

(Mags)

For years Mags had been struggling with 'mental illness' and on seven separate occasions she had gone into hospital looking for help. She had taken 'any number' of different prescribed tablets and seen many psychiatrists and yet, during all that time, 'hope had never occurred to me before!' In fact ineffective professional help had inexorably become part of her despair. Now, within the space of 2 hours, there was hope, a hope that beckoned her. Hope, felt deeply within her body, contained a new story of possibility, which rallied her spirit, tentatively offering and inviting a new direction.

The story Mags heard from the young woman who was a complete stranger with no professional qualifications was a story about recovery 'from such unthinkable and terrifying stuff'. It put Mags's own troubles into perspective, rendering them more manageable and creating the beginnings of empowerment. Witnessing this young woman's recovery opened up the possibility that Mags too could recover. Over the next week her hopeful feelings began to consolidate, thus allowing the birth of new hopeful thoughts which in turn positively affected her behaviour, steering her back towards this potential well of hope:

> I felt, you know I'll go next week, so I went. I wasn't sure exactly what I expected. I wasn't even capable of thinking that far ahead, because I had nearly ended it. I was just struggling from day to day at this stage. I felt I was getting something out of it but I couldn't quite say what. It started with hope.
> (Mags)

Arthur Frank (1995) and Mikhail Bakhtin (1973) both suggest that human growth involves dialogical processes which occur at many different levels of our human existence. It takes time for deeply felt physical sensations, such as terror or hope, which are spontaneous responses to the behaviour of other people, to be translated into meaningful thoughts which can then direct behaviour. In keeping with these ideas it appears that at the early stage of recovery Mags, like many others, could not articulate what the promise of hope would be. Hope was first experienced within her body as a response to the story of the young woman who 'looked a million dollars', but it required the passage of time before she could discover or construct a meaning from that feeling. This hopeful feeling encouraged her to go back to the meeting the following week.

In another interview, Frances spoke about the resonance of ideas which may well be part of her process of personal transformation. She too experienced an epiphany of hope when she heard a recovery story at her first meeting of GROW. Like Mags, this hopeful story began to resonate within her body, awakening hopeful feelings that slowly converted into hopeful thoughts which over time helped create Frances's road out of emotional distress:

> Someone can say something, you listen and it's gone. When it resonates it not only stays but it does some kind of transformation as well. It can be physical and emotional, everything. It changes, it's not come and gone. I suppose GROW resonated with me all along. It 'called me forth' if you like and it's still doing it.
> (Frances)

Lynn, whose trust in people had been shattered through sexual harassment, found that the group re-instilled a spirit of trust, which was a vital element in restoring her faith in people. This in turn created a context in which she could envisage becoming a long-term member of the group and where she would have time to learn new ways of thinking and behaving in a supportive environment:

> It was, the trustworthiness of the whole thing. People were friends, they weren't enemies, they were helping one another. There is only six of us at it

and I have to say that they're so supportive towards me. And I feel now, it's like an alcoholic, I have to go every week, you know. If that makes any sense to you now.

(Lynn)

Jess described his first meeting with GROW members as 'an encounter with joy', and yet his joy came about through watching another man interacting with the group. This encounter dramatically challenged his worldview, or sense of 'what's what' (Frank 1995:8). The other man, who could have been him, was being encouraged to step out of fear while being praised for having the courage to confront that fear. The group was summoning him to bear witness to his own courage, and that summoning of the other touched Jess. There was also no sense that the group saw being afraid as a sign of weakness. Jess was carrying many doubts about his own courage and his identity as a man, and in witnessing this interaction, it was as though there was an interchangeability of self. Jess was able to see himself as the other young man:

It was so enjoyable. There was one man there around my own age, even a couple of years younger. He was being grilled but he took it on so well. If someone had spoken that way to me I would have said 'You can feck off,' but they weren't talking to me, they were talking to someone else. That was a learning experience, I said to myself 'Jesus, I should be able to do that, I should be able to sit and take that kind of constructive criticism'. But they weren't just criticising now, they were praising him for simple little things like you know for getting outside his front door, because he suffered from agoraphobia. I felt so comfortable inside in that room with these people.

(Jess)

Through witnessing the 'other', who could be him, being simultaneously challenged and supported by the other members of the group, Jess glimpsed new possibilities of who he might become, gaining a sense of hope for a different future. He was placed in what Bakhtin (1973) has called biographical time, a time that is at the cross-section of the past and future, a place that suddenly contains resources in the form of other people. People, who Jess 'just couldn't face being with' suddenly became 'so enjoyable'.

Mathew described how joining a GROW group broke the terror in which he had become trapped and suggested that a GROW group, in reality, became a form of larger self, which helped him to break his isolation and get 'out of my own small self into my bigger self'. Mathew's 'small self', the physical unit of his body which contained his soul or spirit, had been dominated by terrifying feelings which in turn gave birth to terrifying imaginings which led to terrifying behaviour. By bringing his physical body to a mutual-help group he automatically brought his fears and his imaginings, and by so doing he placed his own 'terrified' mind inside a larger mind. Other people in the group could provide him with a range of new and hopeful ideas. Through their own stories they could illustrate how they overcame problems similar to his own. By putting his physical body in the presence of other loving bodies, he made himself open to overt and friendly actions of others who were interested in him as a person. The dominant defining feature of Mathew's previous relationships with others had centered around diagnoses of bipolar disorder and schizophrenia. He had experienced others as 'not interested in me only my symptoms'. In the GROW group he met others who wanted to know him as a valued person and wanted to hear his unique story. Once they knew this story, which included living in a terrifying world of 'mythical and strange thinking', they were able to help him learn how to manage these thoughts and successfully control his behaviour. Members of the group would also refer him to different parts of the GROW program and select a 'short story or script', such as the following two quotes, that would help sustain him in between the meetings.

> Feelings are not facts, between a feeling and a fact there is always some at least implicit thought.
>
> (GROW 2001:14)

> A lot of the thoughts that trouble us are nothing but the raw material of our instinctive nature worked into fearful or wishful shapes by a spontaneous imagination. They are not ours in any personal sense and none of them becomes ours except those which we personally appropriate by consenting and choosing to keep them.
>
> (GROW 2001:29)

The idea that recovery involved becoming part of a larger social body is so simple and yet so profound. It represents a huge act of faith, an act of surrender and an acknowledgement of the need of help from others. It is an intentional stepping from a place of lonely alienation into a welcoming social body and a meaningful connection with other people.

Concluding comments

Participants' accounts suggested that deciding to become part of a GROW group often involved an intense internal struggle and frequently only came about through deep despair or the active encouragement of others. Many people reported experiencing very powerful 'somatic stories' of hope, friendship and belonging as a result of attending their first GROW meeting. From the different descriptions of people's early experiences it is clear that the same inter-related dialogical processes that had progressively steered people into 'a place of terror' could also play a part in healing. Whereas feelings of terror and mistrust had given rise to hostile patterns of thinking which in turn led to a desire to isolate from others, now attractive feelings of acceptance, hope, warmth and belonging allowed new thoughts to emerge, thoughts which were full of promise and contained many new possibilities. These thoughts drew individuals towards increasing levels of warm interaction and encouraging involvement with trustworthy others. The experience of being embedded within a larger social body, which included overtly loving others, enabled each person to begin the process of overcoming the alien voices of self-hatred, mistrust, and doubts about the possibility of having a meaningful future. To decide to join a GROW group took a lot of courage; it was an act of faith and it was rewarded by encouragement and acceptance from the other members. The fact that other members of the group had also struggled with difficulties brought with it the comforting realisation that mental distress or 'mental illness' is something that happens to people as an outcome of living, bringing with it a sense of power.

Note

1 The GROW program includes friendly help in a list of tranquillisers which also includes hospital, professional guidance, friendly help, a person's developing resources and a positive life philosophy (GROW 2001:8).

References

Bakhtin, M. 1973. *Problems of Dostoevsky's poetics*, Ann Arbor, MI, Ardis Publishing.
Frank, A. 1995. *The wounded storyteller: Body, illness, and ethics*, Chicago, University of Chicago Press.
GROW 2001. *Program of growth maturity*, Sydney, GROW Publications.

9 A time of healing

The healing power of reciprocal relationship

As time went on you sort of make friends in the group, you realise other people have problems and some of them a lot worse than you, and some of them maybe not as bad, but they're all bad to the person that has them. But the support was great as we got to settle in and get to know people. Everyone supports each other and that's huge. Part of the support is encouragement, encouragement to change, and then the affirmation with tasks or testimonies or whatever. Affirmation is very important.

(Vicky)

As participants settled into regular membership of their GROW group they began to be drawn into a number of healing and reciprocal forms of relationship. Mathew's suggestion, that each group was in fact a larger social self, was reinforced as people described finding themselves cocooned within a benign social womb, where nutrients of recovery, such as hope, courage, acceptance, warmth and compassionate understanding were readily available. Receiving and giving friendship, bearing witness to one another's distress, believing in each other's deep resilience and resourcefulness were all part of the recovery process. Participants became involved in a network of relationships in the wider GROW community and were encouraged to take legitimate risks as they moved away from distress and isolation and began to take responsibility for their own recovery.

Experiencing friendship as a reciprocal relationship

Friendship was repeatedly mentioned as the medium through which seeds of hope, joy, encouragement and a sense of personal value were nurtured. Kenneth Boulding sees friendship as transcending the limitations of being human. Friendship is part of 'a theology of creation'; friends encourage each other 'to let go of life draining images and roles imposed on human beings by social and cultural expectations' (Boulding 1956:31). Friendliness, initially experienced as an outpouring of warmth and unconditional welcome, created a context within which people could begin to trust, feel safe and become hopeful about the future. Being consistently subjected to overt acts of friendship appeared to create a channel through which personal resources, such as hope, courage, self-control, wisdom, acceptance and love, were transferred from one person to another within the nurturing womb of the group. Friendship enabled people to experience a sense of belonging and helped them realise that it was possible to begin a process of positive change with the overt help of caring and trustworthy others:

> I got hope and began to open up. One of the lines [from the GROW program] that's stuck in my mind all through it and still does is 'you alone can do it but you can't do it alone' and that very much stuck in my mind, you know, I thought well I can do this [recover], but I can't do it on my own, I need help.
>
> (Penny)

> It was the friendship it was the closeness of having six or seven other people that talk to you, and these people had troubles of their own. They encouraged me to do things I couldn't have done on my own, like get on a bus or go to the cinema or take part in 12-step work.
>
> (Pat)

Within the group, friendship that at first was uni-directional soon became reciprocal. Claire's story illustrates this. Early on all she can do is be there in her pain. Nothing is asked or expected of her. Soon, however, Claire joins others in reaching out to a newcomer, a young man who was very nervous about attending the meeting. Recalling the difference in herself she says:

> In the beginning [when I first came] I would try to say little things, but I'd cry, and somebody was always there to rub my arm or put their arm around me . . . now we have a young guy that came into us recently, he suffers with [names the medical diagnosis] and it's amazing how he's come on. It's absolutely amazing how he's come on, because he had a drink problem as well . . . he said the first night he came he couldn't get brave enough to come in and he went to the pub and had a drink to get brave enough. He wouldn't speak, he was shy and everything, and he just blossomed into this very confident young man now and he's off the drink a few weeks and we encourage him. We give him a clap and you know, things like that. He always says the one thing he looks forward to is Tuesday night, it's GROW night.
>
> (Claire)

Claire's experience in the group represents a live and compassionate drama. In scene one, she dared to reveal her own brokenness and vulnerability, and this was met with expressed acts of compassion. Then, in scene two, she was called to become a vehicle of compassion for another, a young man who had joined the group.

Peter contrasts the very positive experience of being among a bunch of people honestly striving to overcome problems collaboratively with the traditionally hierarchical and distant relationships that exist within health or education.

> There is something mystical about this realisation of how we are inter-connected. We are all unique but we have these common struggles. We can have a positive effect on each other. It is very different to the whole doctor–patient, teacher–student thing of the more educated person trying to pass on wisdom. It reminds me of the bible saying 'where two or more are gathered'.
>
> (Peter)

Friendship within the group also managed to transcend barriers of age. For example, Peter, a young man of 18 years of age, found he could relate very well to an elderly lady he met in the group:

> Mary was talking about having this paranoid notion that people were always talking about her. And I was having the same thoughts. We connected. I was the youngest at 18 [years of age] and I was connecting with this 76-year-old woman, the oldest there.
>
> (Peter)

Friendships also transcended gender with men and women interacting as fellow humans. This was particularly important to people who had been sexually abused and felt vulnerable. For Vicky, being able to have ordinary friendships with men was something her possessive and violent husband had expressly forbidden.

> It was good to make friends with men and women. I wouldn't have been allowed to meet men. It was quite strange it felt quite awkward at first. I felt like a bold child. Now having men friends is not a big issue.
>
> (Vicky)

Compassionate witness of each other's story

An important part of the reciprocity of friendship involved compassionately wit-nessing each other's stories. Just as important as finding a solution to a problem was having a safe place where it was ok to have problems. All the people in this study had the common experience of never being able to tell someone or hav-ing nobody to listen to their experiences of trauma. GROW was a place where people could learn to tell whatever aspects of their story they chose without fear of consequences.

> The first level where GROW helped me was the idea that I'm going to have a safe environment to actually share some of my so-called 'madness'.
>
> (Charlie)

That two hours every week was a real sanctuary, a great resource. That I could go in and just be there in a safe environment and just talk a little bit was like lifting a great burden.

(James)

Tom found huge relief in just being able to discuss, in a confidential space, issues that he had been bottling up for years:

They said, well in here, you can say whatever you like, and it's confidential, so I was able to talk about some issues. And I found then, I said 'there's great relief here, I actually can talk about some things'. One of the things that made me actually feel the very best though, was feeling the connection, the friendship.

(Tom)

Rappaport (2005:796) suggests that telling personal stories creates meaning and has powerful effects on human behaviour, as 'they tell us not only who we are, who we have been, but who we can be[come]'. For Mathew, telling his story was transforming because he gained a genuine sense that the group was interested in getting to know him as a person rather than his symptoms:

It [telling my story] was healing because people knew what I felt, they empathised, they understood, they were interested.

(Mathew)

Vicky described how 'telling the untellable' to her group helped her come to terms with many confused and destructive feelings and begin to actively take part in her own recovery.

[Telling my story in] GROW allowed me to recognise my feelings. It gave me permission. All my life I have had this anger thing . . . it is wrong to lose your temper, it is selfish to say no. GROW was a safe place to say things and to learn that it is OK to say no or to get angry if a situation warrants it. It began to make me feel differently. I felt a different person because I could now talk about issues. I started to look at my better points and strengths and how I can change things.

(Vicky)

Being listened to and being believed allowed Vicky to own and take control of her feelings, rendering them increasingly manageable. It enabled her to start leaving her emotional prison by changing her thinking and behaviour. In this way she became an agent in her own healing as new ways of thinking and acting opened up new possibilities.

For David, hearing other people's stories validated his struggle so far. At one time he had become suicidal, unable to contemplate a worthwhile future, and now he could begin to build a hopeful picture of what recovery might mean to him.

> Everybody was kind of very friendly, their testimonies gave me hope with the ideas that I'd struggled for years and [a belief] that my struggle was somehow worthwhile, that was the initial, initial effect. And, it helped me with things like loneliness, I became friends with the people in the group.
>
> (David)

Witnessing other people's stories broke bonds of isolation and difference, opening the way for participants to tell their own stories. Paul, who had committed a serious crime and had been in a series of prisons and secure units, had never heard anyone else's story and had thought his own was unique.

> The testimonies, I found that really valuable because I realised that there were a lot of other people who had been through traumas. Like everybody tells their story slightly differently as well, some people you can detect that they don't really want to talk about their story or exactly what happened, so they kind of skirt around it, but still you can get the jist of their experience. And it was those testimonials that I found very valuable in helping me definitely. They made it possible for me to tell my own.
>
> (Paul)

Richard described how hearing the stories of others gave him tremendous hope:

> Well I'll tell you what I found, I mentioned the testimonies, the testimonies were immense, a high, I had lost hope, I really had lost hope, I thought I was on some sort of a slippery slope and I was just in decline, I had been in decline for years, I had found myself just getting more depressed and less able to cope and so on and so forth. And here now were stories of recovery, and not just stories, but the people who had recovered, they were there in front of me you know, it was wonderful.
>
> (Richard)

Being challenged to change and take risks

Legitimate risk taking has been identified as an important part of recovery. Clinical psychologist Geoff Shepherd suggests that 'risk taking needs to be differentiated into risks that must be minimised (self-harm, harm to others) and risks that people have a right to experience', which are necessary for growth and development (Shepherd *et al.* 2008:8). While membership in GROW began with the acceptance and support of the person as they were, as they began to tell their stories of suffering, it soon evolved into a supportive challenge to change, which involved taking positive risks. Challenge and positive risk taking were carefully tailored to each person's current stage of recovery. Each challenge carried with it a reasonable amount of positive risk and became a systematic stepping stone to personal growth and greater levels of life participation.

Lynn, whose faith in people had been badly shaken by her experience of sexual harassment, was able to contemplate risking social involvements.

> The group gave me the task of taking time out for myself. I am now thinking of going on one of the region's social days out, this is something I just couldn't have thought of doing before.
>
> (Lynn)

Positive risk taking suggestions within the group were always accompanied by endorsement, which sometimes became a necessary incentive.

> To get endorsement from the group was great. The one thing I was lacking was endorsement for anything. I wasn't giving myself any. If I hadn't the group I wouldn't have done my practical tasks.[1]
>
> (James)

Challenge involved building trust within the group. A challenge could awaken negative feelings that took time to come to terms with. These feelings could arise when attempting an accepted and agreed practical task at the weekly meeting. For Sue, having the support of another group member who she trusted empowered her to take positive risks even in the face of strong negative feelings:

> [My task] was to leave the house, just walk to the edge of the estate. It was terrifying to begin with. The very first thing I actually did was go for a walk with somebody. I always remember, it was a beautiful September morning and I did the walk and after I had a cup of coffee, and I thought 'I don't believe I actually did that'. It was somebody else having faith in me that 'Yes you can do this'.
>
> (Sue)

Sometimes the group directly challenged and supported people to look at key relationships or attitudes to others which could be very distressing. Jess, who had been sexually and physically abused, was challenged by the group to let go of his anger. Although at first he found it impossible to contemplate, through a mixture of support and challenge, Jess came to a new understanding which liberated him from his toxic hatred and futile lust for revenge.

> When I had explained the abuse thing and how I wanted to kill the bastard, Mary said 'why don't you let go and let God'. And I just sat there and said please (I didn't say this to her it was in my head) 'You didn't listen to me you know.' It wasn't just the night watchman, it was the Christian Brothers the way they treated us. I hated all of them. I remember sitting there one night at home and it was like a light came on, you know, to 'Let go and let

God'. It had nothing to do with God, it had nothing to do with whether Mary believed in God or not, it was to do with me finding some way of getting the pressure off.

(Jess)

The value of having a GROW group to support and endorse professional help was also apparent. When Mags was encouraged by a new, young psychiatrist to risk going on holidays, the group's ready endorsement of Dr D's suggestion provided real grounds for confidence that encouraged Mags to take the risk. The group was saying 'we believe in you' and so she 'dared' to travel:

And then she [Psychiatrist] said, 'Now I won't be able to see you for a week or two because I'll be on holiday.' and I said 'Oh lovely. Where are you going and everything?' and she said 'And where are you going?' and I said 'Well I have holidays coming up but I'm not going anywhere as usual and I might go home'. 'I wouldn't recommend that' she said, she thought that [going back to her original home] was part of the problem. But she said 'Where have you ever dreamed of going?' and I said 'I'd love to go to the States!' and she said 'Why don't you?' So I hummed and hawed and I made a whole lot of negative responses and she said think about it and look into it. So then I went to the group (GROW) and I said would I take it as a task, you know, to go on a holiday somewhere and of course I got 110% support, go for it. It wasn't that long afterwards, I went to America alone. It was a great experience and you know the combination of the group and that. When I came back I felt I certainly I'm a long way on. I began to really find my feet, after doing the States, I wasn't as scared of a recurrence or a relapse, definitely not as scared.

(Mags)

Taking responsibility for own recovery

As people began to recover they came to realize that their mental health and recovery were primarily their own responsibility, not that of their doctor or the mental health team. It became clear they had to learn how to deal with their thoughts and feelings rather than expecting medication to do this for them. Taking responsibility involved many areas of life, such as learning techniques for relaxation, learning how to concentrate when thoughts went into a state of panic or confusion, or learning how to act in a healthy manner even when their feelings were protesting loudly. Kate was in a group for many months when she realized she had to take responsibility for her anxious body rather than relying solely on medication:

It started to dawn on me that neither the doctor nor the pills were going to effect a cure. The penny dropped, I had to do my part . . . Quietening my physical self, listen to my body, to my heart beat, try and get in touch with me.

(Kate)

Helen realised that her attitude towards her family was something for which she must take responsibility. She became aware that constantly harping on about their shortcomings and avoiding their good points was keeping her in a 'negative space' and not helping her mental health. Once she realized this it became relatively easy to change:

> When I was still fairly sick the first piece [of the GROW book] that was quoted to me was 'responsibility'. The bit that struck me was 'no matter how we came to be sick, it's our own responsibility to become well' and this blaming really struck me because, at the time, I was terribly negative and if I got the ear of another adult, I would start giving out non-stop about my family and it was too negative. We do have problems and we always have them, but there was also a good side and there still is a good side to my family. I never gave them that recognition, and it was unbalanced, and at best it was rude to a relative stranger to take them over and vent my, my feelings on them, which is what I had been doing. This bit on blaming struck me and I said well I can stop this, if it's only out of courtesy to other people and the fact that it is a more rational way of going on. So that insight was very helpful and it worked very quickly. I didn't ever struggle with it, it kind of convinced me almost immediately.
>
> (Helen)

Peter reported how GROW helped him take responsibility for his life habits and relationships with other people.

> GROW was a means of learning to connect with other people, to communicate with other people, so I could learn better to understand other people. It was also a means to learn to be able to express myself. I began to look after my diet and avoid stimulants. The [importance] of a regular sleep pattern was something it took me a long time to learn.
>
> (Peter)

Jess began to take responsibility for his emotions, learning that he could choose to take control of his anger, that at various times in his life, took control of him.

> If I sit there in anger with someone, eventually I am learning to think you know ah come on stop yourself, you're just being silly here, you're just being stupid and it's an anger, it's an emotion, find out what's really causing the trouble and deal with it.
>
> (Jess)

Recovery and the reality of setbacks

Many people who have written personal accounts of their own recovery are clear that healing and recovery are not linear processes and will involve many setbacks (Deegan 1995, Maddock and Maddock 2006, Saks 2007). While each person was consistently supported and challenged in their efforts to recover and grow, participants reported that support was particularly valuable during setbacks. For instance, Ruth experienced depression in the midst of her recovery. While she could 'feel nothing', the group provided her with warmth and the promise that if they could recover so could she:

> The depression came back. I could feel nothing, absolutely nothing. It's a horrible thing. I'll never forget the warmness of the meetings. Over the six weeks I heard stories of people who have managed in their lives and the best was, there was a way back.
>
> (Ruth)

Sue experienced a setback after being challenged to take on the leadership role of group recorder. When the role proved too difficult there was no fuss, no labels such as 'failure'. Another member of the group stepped in and took it on until she was ready:

> They asked me to be recorder but I had to do everything perfect (laughing). I wasn't able to do the recording the very first time. I just couldn't do it. So I gave it up and somebody else took it on . . . I came back to be recorder within a year of that. Eventually I became group organiser.
>
> (Sue)

Sue's account shows active support through an ongoing flexibility. The group continued to believe in Sue's ability to perform a leadership role rather than conveying to her the idea that she had failed.

Pat spoke of how, if someone stopped attending a meeting they would be contacted and encouraged rather than forgotten or blamed for not attending:

> The first time I had a relapse, thank God I had the phone anyway, I was getting phone calls, the contacts were being made.
>
> (Pat)

Peter reported how he was supported through a time of crisis, triggered by his decision to withdraw from medication. Another member of the group who was now living successfully without the help of 'lifelong' medication was able to offer support and moderate the intensity of the return of feelings of terror (exacerbated by Peter's worried parents) by advising a slow withdrawal from medication:

> My instinct was that meds didn't suit me. I stopped taking [names antipsychotic medication], which meant I couldn't sleep. I thought, I'll stop the lot so I decided to stop. My parents were very worried. They met with someone in the group [from GROW] who had successfully come off medication. I agreed to talk to her. She said don't go off everything at once so I decided to

stay on [names another drug], but came off all the rest. I was very close to going back into hospital it was one of those crucial moments in my life.

(Peter)

GROW as an extended family

Several people used the term 'family' to describe their experience of GROW. For them, especially those who had been traumatized by abuse and neglect while living within their family of origin, GROW provided them with a second chance to find the kind of intense love and protection that might reverse the damaging effects of traumatic pasts. Peg, who had been an extraordinarily anxious child and periodically had long periods where she refused to attend school, described GROW in this way.

GROW was a little bit like being born into a different family, being given another chance. Obviously I wouldn't blame my parents you know, for that [her anxiety], because they were only young with seven kids, they were doing the best they could, but [through GROW] I learned a lot.

(Peg)

For Richard, GROW was a family that provided him with love and understanding.

I was loved back to health. The time people gave me when I was ill, the effort people made for me, it was wonderful. Yea, and that 'you can recover', that belief that 'you can recover, and that you are valuable'. And you know 'the bad in you can be remedied, and the good can grow'. But the lady who was, the organiser of the Group at the time, she used to contact me on a daily basis, just for a few minutes on the telephone. Now I found that to be very very healing, that there was somebody who actually understood, because I would have to say my family didn't understand, they hadn't suffered from depression, they didn't know what clinical depression was and all that there. And here I had all these people who did understand you know.

(Richard)

For Claire, the group, as family, provided a place where she could recover from the tragic double suicide of her son and grandson. A relationship with a young man in her group, who she thought of as her son, began a healing process and a way back to life:

This young man, he's in his 30s now. He was only 2 years married and his marriage breaks up, this is a man who'd buried his brother by suicide and had a pretty bad life as a young child. He'd lost his mother. She died when he was only twelve. And we were sort of very close because to me he's the son I lost and I was the mother he lost.

(Claire)

By caring for and responding to this young man, who was so terribly in need, as the son she had lost, Claire found a way to begin to live and hope again, and her own life was enriched.

The concept of 'GROW as family' soon led to a much wider involvement within an extending GROW community. Julian Rappaport (1988:8) described GROW groups as 'the glue which holds a whole community together'. From the very beginning of membership, people reported being actively encouraged to make contact outside the weekly meeting and to become friends with other members of their group. Penny recalls how a friend she made in GROW supported her after she was discharged from hospital and vulnerable:

> If I felt down and maybe was crying here [at home] on my own . . . and if I rang Madge crying, Bobby [Madge's partner] would be in, in five minutes. She lives a couple of miles away and he'd bring me out [to Madge] and wouldn't bring me back maybe 'til l0 ten o'clock at night, and I'd come back laughing.
>
> (Penny)[2]

Some participants who attended social events involving members of different GROW groups described how this led to the discovery of new or hidden talents and gifts. Peg was a gifted singer but was crippled with fear of singing in front of people. When she attended an informal social evening in the home of another group member she overcame that fear with the support of friends:

> We had twelfth step[3] in M's house and I sang one [song] with the lights out. This was great growth for me. I suddenly realized, I could actually do things. I discovered I could sing [without fear].
>
> (Peg)

Singing later became a vehicle through which Peg extended her social networks outside GROW, singing at church, joining a folk choir and visiting a women's prison to sing.

A major social event in the GROW calendar is the community weekend attended by up to 300 GROW members from different groups. In the same way that attending a first GROW meeting could require effort, attending social events often meant overcoming significant barriers of fear. Pat's interview revealed a lifetime of being bullied by children, by teachers and by managers at work. This may well explain his being 'terrified' at the thought of spending a whole weekend in the company of unknown other people. Instead of being bullied and humiliated, Pat discovered fellowship, people shook his hand and he [his fear] was 'blown away':

> I went on the weekend and I was fecking terrified, but several GROWers came and I was brought down in a car. I was absolutely blown away. I said 'what in the name of God'. It was great just to see so many people with difficulties and friendship and people shaking hands with you, a fellowship.
>
> (Pat)

For Cathy, who had been swamped by feelings of anxiety, the weekend was a reminder of good things that had made her life valuable when she was a child. To be reconnected with singing and dancing was a turning point towards freedom.

> There was a sense of freedom. Friday night was a very relaxing thing. We all sat and it reminded me of when I was very young and having family get-togethers and singing, curled up on a chair and laid back. And I just sang because everybody was singing and it was like this great freedom.
>
> (Cathy)

For Helen, attending a weekend softened her view of other people, changing her behaviour towards her family. It was also the start of her extending her social networks outside GROW by attending other social events and groups (like Comhaltas[4] and the Irish Country-Women's Association, ICA):

> I was delighted with it [the weekend]. It was very friendly and warm and encouraging and refreshing. I was delighted, and it was social as well, and then that Christmas I started thinking about my little nieces and nephews and I softened towards people and because of the confidence I got socialising in GROW, I started going out to other things.
>
> (Helen)

Richard, who is a talented musician, found his first GROW weekend to be both educational and enjoyable. One of the workshops helped him understand his feelings of anxiety in a non-threatening way, and the atmosphere of fun and dancing encouraged him to take out his guitar and sing:

> I remember going to a weekend and thinking I want to get back here again. Gertrude [a seasoned GROW leader] did her workshop about stress and the wheels of a car. I was riveted thinking this explains things so well. It also encouraged me with music in front of people. It was lovely to watch some of the dancers. It was a complete escape and a place of great fun.
>
> (Richard)

Without attending the weekend, Richard would have missed the workshop. Later he reported 'extending his social network' by going back to full-time study. However, like all the other participants, it was the nature of the weekend that impressed him most. Music, dance, warmth, friendship and laughter were continually mentioned as the most healing part of extending social networks.

Concluding comments

As soon as new members had settled into their weekly GROW meeting, they were invited to become involved in a number of reciprocal activities which became instrumental in their recovery. After receiving abundant friendship from others they now began to actively befriend others in the group. They began to share their own stories of recovery and progress as well as bearing witness to those of others. They began to accept challenges and risk making small personal changes in the direction of recovery and to endorse others for doing the same. With this came a growing realisation that recovery was partly about taking personal responsibility and developing healthy ways to live. People described being supported through inevitable setbacks that were part of their recovery and being able to offer similar support to others. They suggested that being in GROW was in effect like being part of an alternative family which offered them a second chance at life. People provided examples of becoming increasingly involved in a widening network of friendly relationships that are part of the wider GROW community. It was as David Konstan (1997:108–109) suggests, 'friendship dance[d] round the world proclaiming to us all to wake up for happiness'. Through friendship, people began to be liberated from the toxic identity of 'mental patient' or 'hopeless other', and their terror and isolation began to be transformed into a healing and reciprocal belonging, creating what Schweitzer and Lemke (1998) called 'a brotherhood of suffering'.

Notes

1 Each person in a GROW group identifies a goal to be achieved in the week ahead. This is known as taking on a practical task. The following week each person is asked what progress they have made with their task and they are endorsed for efforts made irrespective of how well they have achieved their goal'.
2 This kind of informal interacting perhaps presents a nightmare for health and safety legislation but is indicative of the necessary risks involved in recovery.
3 The term 'twelve-step' or 'twelfth-step work' refers to any interactions between GROW members that take place outside the formal GROW structures.
4 Comhaltas is an organization that promotes Irish music and dancing.

References

Boulding, K. E. 1956. *The image: Knowledge in life and society*, London and Ann Arbor, MI, Paperbacks.
Deegan, P. 1995. Coping with recovery as a journey of the heart. *Psychiatric Rehabilitation Journal*, 19, 91–97.
Konstan, D. 1997. *Friendship in the classical world*, Cambridge, Cambridge University Press.
Maddock, M. & Maddock, J. 2006. *Soul survivor: A personal encounter with psychiatry*, Sheffield, Asylum Books.
Rappaport, J. 1988. *The evaluation of GROW in the USA and its significance for community and mental health.* GROW National Seminar, Sydney.
Rappaport, J. 2005. Community psychology is (thank God) more than science. *American Journal of Community Psychology*, 35, 231–238.
Saks, E. R. 2007. *The center cannot hold: My journey through madness*, New York, Hyperion.
Schweitzer, A. & Lemke, A. B. 1998. *Out of my life and thought: An autobiography (1931)*, Baltimore, MD, John Hopkins University Press.
Shepherd, G., Boardman, J. & Slade, M. 2008. *Making recovery a reality*, London, Sainsbury Centre for Mental Health.

10 A time of healing

Leadership, choosing 'goodness', new identities and resilience

Well the role of the [GROW group] organiser is a big responsibility, so it was a big challenge. You are the key holder. The main task is to have the room ready, and then if anyone new comes in introduce and make them feel welcome, try to do everything you can, because I know myself when I came to the first GROW meeting I was very nervous. I said nothing for 3 or 4 weeks.

(Danny)

While friendship was the principle medium through which people were initially nurtured and empowered in their recovery, leadership also played a very significant role. Within mutual help, leadership is a reciprocal relationship, a function shared by everyone rather than being provided by members of an elite hierarchy who expect others to follow unquestioningly. After initially experiencing acts of leadership from others, such as receiving a warm welcome, having your story listened to and witnessed by a caring other or having the meeting facilitated by an 'ordinary' person, participants described how they were supported to develop a wide range of leadership skills themselves. Participants also identified striving to be good as central to their recovery. Being good did not mean being a 'good patient' or blindly following a prescribed care regime, but being actively involved in exploring healthy lifestyle habits in order to master unruly feelings, thoughts and behaviours. Becoming actively involved in leadership and striving to do what was 'good', in the context of supporting yet challenging others, led participants to the awakening of personal resilience and the discovery of new and positive identities.

The key role of leadership

While taking responsibility for one's own recovery began with learning to care for oneself, it soon extended to taking responsibility for the quality of the GROW meeting and subsequently for the wider GROW community. Taking responsibility in this way meant becoming involved in leadership. GROW describes leadership as 'love showing the way' (GROW, Undated:31), a shared activity that is 'good' for both the individual and the organisation. In the first few months of attending meetings, people learned how to tell their story, give a report on progress, identify a practical task or facilitate a meeting. All these involvements are acts of leadership, all involve taking responsibility for the group as a whole and all bring with them direct benefits. Many participants described how leadership positively challenged their habitually negative and powerless self-image, providing seeds for a new and positive identity as well as affirming latent abilities. Leadership might begin with something as simple as making tea or washing up. Mags began her contribution in the following way:

> After about 6 or 7 weeks I did something that I would never have done. I offered to make tea. I just kept saying to myself, if they [other members] can do it, I can. Another week I helped with the wash-up and the other person started to chat to me, very ordinary stuff like the weather and the news, and I felt safe in it.
>
> (Mags)

For James, leadership involved learning how to share his story and take part in discussions in which his own lived experience could be of help to others:

> For me general chit-chat was like a military operation. I had everything planned out what I was going to say. And I needed practice at listening to general conversation and being emphatic and also practice at partaking in conversation. So I found it good to be able to do that to be able to give opinions and advise from your own personal experience.
>
> (James)

After 6 months of attendance, a period in which new members learned the basic leadership skills involved in holding a weekly meeting, people reported being invited to take on formal leadership roles, such as becoming a group organiser or recorder,[1] something which many people found to be both challenging and rewarding.

For Richard, taking on the responsibility of becoming an Organiser provided a way to escape a self-made prison of perfectionism:

> A liberating idea [from GROW] is that it's OK to do things badly at the beginning. I was asked to be organiser and thought I couldn't, then I thought it would be ridiculous not to do it, just because I couldn't do it perfectly. GROW gave me permission to have a go at things.
>
> (Richard)

For Nan, it affirmed her value. People must be able to see qualities in her that she could not see in herself, giving her a basis for self belief:

> I went every week to my meeting, I was hanging on for dear life. After a few months I was leading a meeting and after a short time, I think a year God

bless them they asked me would I become organiser. And of course this was so unusual to me because I couldn't believe, I didn't believe in myself. They obviously saw something in me that they liked.

(Nan)

Jess, who had joined GROW when he was feeling suicidal and who also had little sense of his personal value, felt hugely proud about being asked to become the organiser of his group:

I remember M asking me would I accept the challenge of becoming organiser of the group and I remember inside, while I wasn't able to express, was this huge feeling, it was like my heart got bigger inside in my chest. I've had positions of authority in the army and none of them meant as much as being asked to be organiser of the Thursday night group.

(Jess)

Perhaps taking on responsibility for the group through a formal leadership role had such a deep and healing effect on Jess because it was in direct contrast to the leadership of Jess's place of work, the army. Within this context, leadership is always part of an 'ascribed hierarchy' equated with status, rank and qualifications. In contrast, Jess saw this request as affirmation of his positive qualities as a human being and his ability to work compassionately with others.

As people became proficient in leadership attached to the successful running of the weekly meeting, many became actively involved in leadership at a more regional and even national level. Involvement in the 'bigger picture' of GROW included activities such as supporting other groups, giving talks in schools or joining the regional or national team. The weekly GROW meeting served as a place where people learned and practised leadership skills in parallel with work on their own recovery. Overcoming fears connected to leadership outside the sheltered weekly meeting gave Kate a sense of excitement and enthusiasm for what might lie ahead, and for Pat, it eradicated a sense of stigma associated with his label of 'mental illness'.

We started travelling to other groups and realised God we aren't the only one. I went to a leadership meeting. Getting a bigger picture was extremely helpful. It was terrifying at first, but there was part of me that was really excited because I was so isolated at the time, I was so isolated at the time that to want to go anywhere was a huge new thing to me. I had completely disconnected myself from so many people and so many situations, I had lost touch with all of my friends. So for me to even, even have a glimmer of interest in anything was remarkable. So going to these things was beginning to generate in me a little bit of interest. I wouldn't use the word 'enthusiasm' because I didn't feel that for a long time.

(Kate)

I would go out and give testimonies out in groups from time to time, R [names a GROW employee] brought me out to a group recently, and I put leaflets on the buses. And I have even worked in the office voluntary. There is a stigma attached to 'mental illness', but as I say it is a badge of honour for me now to be able to share my story and help others.

(Pat)

Choosing to be a good ordinary person

The word 'goodness' is defined as 'virtue, excellence, benevolence' (Chambers 2010:415), and it was a recurring theme in the narratives of the participants. Philosophers such as Aristotle (384–322 BC), Thomas Aquinas (1274 AD) and Immanuel Kant (1724–1804 AD) and all major religions have long associated goodness with the pursuit and acquisition of health and happiness. One of GROW's first principles advises

> do whatever ordinary and good people do, and avoid whatever ordinary and good people avoid' and to 'never say I can't, if the thing in question is an ordinary and a good thing. Do the ordinary thing you fear, do the ordinary thing that repels you.
>
> (GROW 2001:7–32)

The promised benefits, according to GROW, of striving to be good and developing right habits of thinking and acting are that 'feelings will get better as . . . habits of thinking and acting get better' and that 'special abilities will develop in harmony if [the person's] aim is to be a good ordinary human being' (GROW 2001:10–11).

Participants' accounts included many descriptions of striving 'to be a good ordinary human being' and confirmed the healing effects of adopting this as a life strategy. Richard described how GROW, as a practical theology, began to influence his life choices. He spoke of a number of instances when he had based his actions on the concept of 'doing the ordinary and good thing', pushing himself to go out and meet people when he desperately wanted to hide away, learning to overcome a fear of singing in front of other people and becoming a group organiser. All these actions became an important part of his recovery.

> It's funny, GROW has become very much a part of my theology, the idea of goodness. I could put it that way. You know the whole thing is that 'do the good and right thing' you know, for yourself, or for somebody else. You know the good and right thing is essentially the loving choice, you know, and if God is love, then that is God prompting us to do the good and right thing, and by learning to do the ordinary and good thing we find that life becomes more manageable.
>
> (Richard)

The GROW program contains a number of references to God as being a healing resource, and while belief in God is optional within GROW, some participants reported how the word 'God' became synonymous with the word 'goodness' and in this way God [as goodness] became a very practical part of their inner healing. Jess had rejected formalised religious practices, and yet the idea of God as goodness became a mainstay of his recovery:

> At the start I struggled with the God thing. Changing the word 'God' to 'good' really made sense for me. To believe in the good was huge, it has helped me overcome an awful lot.
>
> (Jess)

Consistently striving to be good, either by choosing to overcome personal obstacles in life or by increasingly becoming involved in the 'good ordinary process' of helping others, provided people with a systematic road to recovery. By using the idea of goodness as a signpost for their daily actions, participants began to change. For James, a developing belief in the power of goodness through his own personal work, through the nurturing actions of others and through developing leadership skills, slowly brought about a change in his belief system. His changing outlook enabled him to increasingly open himself up to the healing power of goodness which helped him escape from a 'place of terror' where the 'devil had been in charge':

> [Previously] I had come to the conclusion that goodness in the world is just a futile effort. The devil is in charge. That was my world view. Then it was explained to me to substitute the word 'God' with the word 'good' and then to look at goodness. I found the more you open yourself up to a particular belief system that's the way your belief system will be. If you look for bad you will find bad in the world. You have to feed the good.
>
> (James)

David completely rejected the idea of God but still professed a belief in the power of goodness and in an ethic of good and healthy living. While studying philosophy he had come across Aristotle's idea of ethical living, and this idea resonated with him, enabling him to move away from a nihilistic view where nothing held meaning. By doing what his reason told him was the good thing, rather than what he felt like doing, he began to develop many new healthy habits and began to explore many new and hopeful life possibilities. David after a period of time returned to study and became involved in hill walking, both of which were 'good ordinary things' and both of which began to enrich the quality of his life.

> I was kind of, I suppose I was a nihilist of sorts, by a nihilist I mean someone who just didn't see any hope for anything; I just saw mental illness everywhere. I [now] believe in good in the sense of Aristotle's ethical living in the sense of a good day, in a sense of Aristotle, in the sense of flourishing.
>
> (David)

Throughout these findings, people's narratives consistently indicated the value of having dependable and ongoing support from others. This is often referred to as horizontal spirituality and is basically a belief in each other's ability to change, to grow and to recover. Horizontal spirituality is defined in the GROW program as 'mutual belief – belief in one another, hope for one another and love of one another' (GROW 2001:69). Richard's story illustrates how horizontal spirituality works in practice.

> Another thing that I found was, I didn't realise it at the time, but you know this whole concept of vertical and horizontal spirituality. I remember Patricia giving her testimony, and it was just, it was electrifying because here was somebody who had obviously had a very very very serious 'mental illness', and here I was looking at her, and she was, you know, a fully functioning, a great woman, holding down a responsible job in the community. . . . I was just bowled over by that. The horizontal spirituality was . . . that I couldn't believe in myself, but other people believed in me. And I found that, that belief in me, from other people was great. That belief that 'you can recover, and that you are valuable'. And the bad in you can be remedied, and the good can grow. It meant the world to me that belief.
>
> (Richard)

As they moved further along towards recovery, many participants, such as Nan and Kate, testified that they began to experience internally generated and spontaneous periods of well-being, which made them feel good about themselves and which made them appreciative of the goodness around them:

> I began to feel good about myself. Feeling good about yourself is a wonderful positive energy . . . recovery to me means being happy with life. To appreciate the good in the here and now, enjoy a cup of coffee, to be able to plant a bulb and know there will be a flower in spring.
>
> (Nan)

> The core issue of my problems was with my self esteem. Because I was learning to think more by reason than by feelings and imagination, I was getting long periods where I was feeling good. And those periods were giving me the opportunity then to change my thinking, to change my behaviour, I was getting a break from the intense feelings of anxiety that I was experiencing and my thinking was becoming clearer and my plan, the plan was starting to form about where I was going and how I was going to go there.
>
> (Kate)

For Frances, whose illegitimate birth had totally undermined any sense that she had a right to be alive, the advice to 'do the ordinary and good thing she feared' became a personal call to become the best person she could. This had a profound effect on her sense of personal value and her belief about why anyone is born.

> That's if I'm the best I can be and I'm not talking about achievements, if I'm the most joyful, the most loving, the most caring, the most that I can be, then God is glorified. You know, why am I on this earth? Why am I here? I remember once reading in a book and it struck me like a rocket, em . . . God does not love you because you are here, but you are here because God loves you.
>
> (Frances)

Frances began to acknowledge that she was someone who had very real gifts and that through developing these gifts she would discover her own path to recovery. Later Frances developed a successful career as a trainer, working first in a mental health context and then within a parish:

> [I discovered] I'm never more alive than when I'm in front of a group . . . at a workshop or something like that. I just come alive there, I come alive in a group . . . I know that's my forte. I knew I have gifts but I wouldn't have believed in them, GROW enabled me to see them.
>
> (Frances)

Many participants described how happiness and an emerging sense of well-being were the by-products of becoming involved in leadership and adopting a life philosophy that involved always striving to be good. This sense of well-being, in turn, began to positively affect the way people viewed themselves, creating glimpses of a new and exciting identity that might lie ahead.

Discovering a new identity

Low self-esteem, a sense of personal powerlessness and the social stigma attached to 'mental illness' were perhaps the defining features of people when they first came to GROW. David had reported that even when his doctor was being pleasant to him he, could not shake the hopelessness that came with the identity of being 'mentally ill'. Kate, Tom and Peter recounted a terrible sense of feeling that they would be 'mental patients' for the rest of their lives and became increasingly pessimistic that anything could change their awful identity. Through involvement in their group, through experimenting with leadership roles and by striving to become 'good people' participants reported a growing sense of a new and positive identity and a realisation of their own worth and ability to change their life situation. Frances's story illustrates this very well.

The main difficulty many people faced when they came to GROW was the 'negative scripts' or identities they had received from a whole range of others and the negative sense of self this engendered over time. Frances was born outside of marriage and was considered illegitimate. One of the definitions of the word 'legitimate' in Chambers dictionary (2010) is 'genuine'. The word 'illegitimate' is not so different etiologically from the word 'in-valid'. By being illegitimate she had been created less than genuine. Illegitimacy had been the socially constructed label and identity, the unasked-for, the unwanted story of her life:

> I had no sense of myself. I didn't know who I was. I had very strong hang ups about being illegitimate. I had learnt a lot of lessons from people in the society in which I lived, from neighbours, from my own family, from my foster family, from children in school, that I was different, that I was less. Even religion entered into it. My overriding feeling was of insecurity and rejection.
>
> (Frances)

This monumental sense of having a hopeless identity was also well illustrated in Cathy's narrative. When she first became hospitalised she was overwhelmed by a sense of hopelessness and stigma which she believed would continue forever:

> So it was a big stigma attached to, and a big realisation, oh my God I'm in hospital. I'm not going to get out. This is me. Locked up . . . I saw myself as mentally ill with no hope.
>
> (Cathy)

Similarly, Kate, who was hospitalised when she was just 22, saw herself as someone with no future. Even though she had a home, a husband and young daughters the identities such as homeowner, wife and mother were decimated by the hopeless identity of 'mental illness'.

> I was mentally ill . . . I was apart from everybody else. I couldn't really talk to people properly. Hope was gone, I'd no hope, I didn't have any sense of anything.
>
> (Kate)

For Frances, Cathy and Kate the negative label of 'mental illness' and 'illegitimacy' completely obscured the possibility of any positive identity, such as daughter, friend, neighbour, and human being. Hence, Frances's statement that 'I didn't know who I was'. For Frances, her family of origin, her foster family, her neighbours, her classmates, even her God reflected the same message: 'You are different!', 'You are less!', 'You have no right to be here!'. These stories and 'authoritative utterances' blocked out any possibility of Frances knowing who she was, other than illegitimate. They also ruled out the possibility of Kate and Cathy creating new alternatives other than the identity of mentally ill, or for Richard, who saw himself as bad, or Vicky, who thought of herself as powerless to forge a positive sense of identity. Once Frances came to GROW she was confronted with the story of another woman who had also been adopted but who was happy with herself and unashamed to speak about her situation.

> I went to my first GROW meeting and a person gave her testimony. It was about being adopted. I was looking at her because I thought she was telling my story. I was looking around as well. I remember going home that night

and saying 'in the name of God why have I carried this?' And I felt so much lighter that I said 'now there is nothing that I need, there is nothing I can't talk about, that was such a block and burden to me'. I really went home ten feet taller that night.

(Frances)

Frances described a moment of social intercourse literally impregnated with the seeds of personal rebirth or transformation of her identity. First, she hears her 'own' story being told by another in a different and positive way. It instantly challenges her beliefs, her thoughts and her sense of self. As sociologist Richard Sennett suggests, 'stories give lives legibility' (Sennett 2007:148). Suddenly, through the lips of another, a new life-giving story is breathed into her. Her own inability to know who she is is swept away. It lifts her spirit; she feels 'ten feet taller'. She does not have to rely solely on the testimony of the storyteller. The faces of others in the group reassure her:

> None of them are running her down. They are completely and emotionally with her. When she finished a lot of affirmation started, and people were saying lots of nice things about her.
>
> (Frances)

There was no sense of rejection by members of the group towards this 'other self' who was 'illegitimate', and not only did she glimpse her own life story differently, but she witnessed a different response from her GROW family. Her story had changed, she had changed and others had changed. After the meeting Frances's reflective response to her experience of that first group was to 'cry out' 'in the name of God why have I carried this?'

Kate and Cathy both found the acceptance of others in a GROW group, and the realisation that other people have struggles too helped them to see beyond their label of mental illness. Sue, whose identity was formed on a belief that nobody could like her, described how expressions of friendship in the group transformed her feelings and thoughts about herself, initiating a process of personal healing and the authoring of a new identity:

> I felt when people got to know me they wouldn't like me. Therefore I didn't want to get to know anybody. When I joined GROW one of the first people I connected with was Liz [pseudonym]. She used to call me her lovely Sue. She used to always give me a great hug at the end of the meeting. And she'd be 'oh you are my lovely Sue'. She was the very first person that awakened that belief that I'm okay and not this horrible person that I had in my head.
>
> (Sue)

Sue is touched by Liz's overt leadership. Touched physically, through the ready warmth of a hug, but also existentially and spiritually by the way Liz calls her by a new name. The words 'My lovely Sue' enable Sue to see herself as she might be, as she already is in the eyes of another, someone who is lovely. She is invited to shed the story of the 'horrible person' she believed herself to be. Liz's behaviour acts as a positive and powerful peripeteia. By physically touching Sue, she removes the fear and stigma that clings to her and which separates her from others. Over time, Liz's repeated words 'Oh you are my lovely Sue' provide a constant and reassuring reference point, a new script or mirror that she can rely on to see a new and emerging version of herself.

Becoming empowered to choose and the birth of resilience

Accounts of increasing progress in their own recovery journey and in leadership within the GROW community depicted the weekly GROW meeting as a place where people were systematically empowered to make choices. Each person reported being encouraged and supported to try out empowering ways of thinking and behaving, even if these new 'life habits' initially precipitated fear or anxiety or triggered a setback. The ongoing practice of choosing to do tasks, such as going for a walk, taking on a leadership role or changing a negative thought, which initially were very challenging, became easier and in the long term provided grounds for confidence for a productive involvement beyond GROW in the much less supportive environment of society. The positive fruits of learning to make choices within GROW brought with them a new language of possibility and with it came internally generated and empowering realisations such as: 'I can do this' (Peter); 'I am allowed to be' (Frances); and 'Others are the same as myself' (James). All of these realisations opened up liberating worlds of possibility and were signs that people who had been beaten down by their experiences of life were becoming resilient. At this point in their recovery people were beginning to cease depending on the encouragement, support and endorsement of other members of the group. Now they were experiencing an enchanting sense of possibility bubbling up from inside themselves, encouraging them to become more and more involved in life.

> I began to sense I needed a challenge.
>
> (Cathy)

> I sensed that even though work was pushing me beyond my limits it was good for me.
>
> (Peter)

> I got a leadership role as class committee person [within the facility where I was working] and I took on the challenge not so much to help my fellow man, but for my own personal growth.
>
> (Mathew)

Slowly people's futures were transformed from something to be dreaded into an exciting and ever present opportunity for change:

> It took 2 to 3 years. I started to relax, people started to get friendlier. The more I relaxed, the more people relaxed around me.
>
> (Tom)

I was able to go out and mix and do different things, go to shows and drive.

(Jack)

Kate described how the constant acceptance of positive challenges opened up the possibility of being able to choose her own kind of future:

All of these things were a challenge . . . every challenge I took on drove me forward a little step. You know and every challenge I took on, maybe made me look at, or want to do something else, so you know what I was learning was creating the foundation for where I went with my life.

(Kate)

Concluding comments

Involvement in many different forms of reciprocal leadership provided an ongoing pathway towards recovery. People learned that recovery and a sense of well-being came about as the by-product of healthy life choices, a process which involved learning to choose to do the ordinary and good thing instead of what they might feel like doing or what might seem to be most expedient. Being involved in leadership and striving to do the good ordinary thing again offered glimpses of new and exciting identities which enabled people to shed feelings of stigma, such as that attached to the label of 'mental illness'. It also opened up a well of resilience, so that the encouragement and support of others gradually gave way to an internal desire to explore life to the full. It was at this point that people began to describe how they successfully joined what Rappaport (2000) called 'pre-existent niches' in society.

Note

1 While leadership is a shared responsibility for all GROW members, progressing and seasoned GROWers are invited to take on various leadership roles while continuing to be ordinary group members. The role of organiser is designed to ensure that meetings are conducted in a safe and standard manner; the recorder is the group's evaluator, filling in a short evaluation of each meeting.

References

Aquinas, T. 1274 AD. *Summa theologica (Fathers of the English Dominican province, Trans.)*, New York, Benziger Brothers.

Aristotle 384–322 BC. *Nicomachean ethics book 1 3:2 defining happiness*, Indianapolis, IN, Cambridge, Hackett Publishing Company Inc.

Chambers 2010. *The Chambers dictionary*, Edinburgh, Harrap Publishers.

GROW 2001. *Program of growth maturity*, Sydney, GROW Publications.

GROW n.d. *GROW program training manual*, Sydney, GROW Publications.

Rappaport, J. 2000. Community narratives: Tales of terror and joy. *American Journal of Community Psychiatry*, 28, 1–24.

Sennett, R. 2007. *The culture of the new capitalism*, New Haven, CT, Yale University Press.

11 A time of growth
Successful social involvements

> Having GROW was good, but having work as well has made my mental health better. Things like hill walking helped me a lot, it is about finding a balance. I think another problem people have is learning to be comfortable with themselves when they are on their own. Going on the odd 8-hour hill walk has made me more confident about being by myself.
>
> (Peter)

While recovery began with a time of healing spent in the weekly meeting of GROW and was nurtured through widening involvements in the larger GROW community, participants all agreed that recovery was greatly enhanced by increased participation in society. Involvement in GROW had facilitated an increasing ability to make choices and take legitimate and courageous risks in the direction of recovery. It had also helped nurture a more positive sense of self and a greater sense of personal agency and resilience to a level that participants were empowered to concentrate on forging greater involvement outside the sheltered environment of the GROW community. Whilst using their GROW group as a base for encouragement and reflective wisdom, people began to explore different challenging social environments. People's accounts provided concrete examples of their increasing involvement in work, education and leisure activities, which represented another phase in their healing and recovery and the beginning of full citizenship.

The healing influence of work

One of the most significant niches of involvement reported by participants was employment. Work, whether paid or unpaid, was important for a number of reasons. For example, Kate and her husband were both unemployed with three small children. After 2 years in GROW, Kate began to feel she was ready to return to work. Returning to work required courage, a spiritual resource that had taken 2 years to 'gather':

> One of the biggest things was returning to work . . . it was the beginning of me taking responsibility and my place back in the world . . . [In GROW] I had

gathered the courage and belief that 'I can do this, indeed I have to do it'. It was necessary that one of us had some work and was earning some money. So I went back and I did a job and it was probably one of the best things that ever happened to me.

(Kate)

Just as being a 'patient' in the hospital had proffered a social script that defined Kate's identity, so did being employed. Being hospitalised represented a belief that Kate had become a danger to 'herself or others' and could not be trusted. By giving her a job and putting her in charge of a 'million dollars' worth of machinery', her employers demonstrated a tangible story of trust. Being involved in the GROW group had provided Kate with reasonable grounds for confidence to trust herself enough to step successfully into that story. While negative memories of the past were still very real, the ongoing experience of employment allowed Kate to sense that they could be overcome. Kate did not wait until she was fully recovered to seek employment; instead, employment and the struggles she encountered, became part of her recovery:

It [the job] was full time and it was a night shift. At the time I wouldn't have left myself in control of flushing the toilet, but they were leaving me in control of a million dollars' worth of machinery and I think 'Jesus if they knew' . . . It was really helpful. I went somewhere for 8 hours and was too busy to think of myself. Though I used to have my moments, I would go out to the loo and close the door and try to breathe and try to get a grip, and I would take my medication because I would still be taking medication at the time. It was about diverting your attention; this job was diverting my attention away from concentrating 24 hours a day on my feelings.

(Kate)

Kate's experience resonates with accounts of other participants. For example, Peter began working in a voluntary capacity with people with an intellectual disability [ID] and found that he no longer had time for the negative thoughts that had habitually haunted him. Having voluntary work changed his idea of himself. He came to recognise that he had a valuable contribution to make to society, especially when working with others who, like him, had been socially marginalised.

In the beginning I wasn't really responsible for anyone I just worked on the farm and spent time with O [names a man with ID]. Then an interesting thing happened a guy who had a role with O crashed his car so I was responsible for O. It worked to my advantage, because I didn't expect it, it just happened. It was a lot of work but it suited me. I couldn't be depressed and spend time thinking negatively. Because of my experience of being hospitalised and on medication I saw myself as a burden [on other people]. Now I was able to contribute, to look after someone, it had a huge impact on my self-esteem.

(Peter)

Similarly, Jack was going through quite a difficult time in his life and found having work distracted him from the daily negativity of his life:

> So I feel better going to work, it's only at home thinking, all these things come to your mind and being in work keeps your mind occupied, it's very important, At the time we had some problems at home, the mother fell sick and we had other losses.
>
> (Jack)

By continually allowing their minds to dwell on themselves, Jack, Kate and Peter were dwelling on the negative stories of the past and current difficulties, which tended to maintain their habitual fearful pattern of emotions and thoughts. Diverting their attention through work made room for the emergence of new stories at many levels. These included new feelings or 'somatic stories' of accomplishment; 'cognitive stories' such as 'I can do this'; 'interpersonal stories' of appreciative acceptance from colleagues and a 'cultural' and 'authoritative story' in the form of an employment contract, monetary reward and being a contributing citizen. So just as terror was seen to spawn other destructive feelings such as hate, rejection or resentment, Kate, Jack and Peter's behaviour was beginning to generate and nurture positive feelings, and they began to exert control over their destiny and to experience agency, which enabled them to continue to re-author their story. During this time of entering the workforce, encouragement and endorsement from their group helped them realize the value of their efforts to be ordinary. Jack in particular felt his group's encouragement was vital to the progress he was making with his life.

> The encouragement was great. You're not inclined to [endorse yourself] you know what I mean, in a sense, you could be doing, doing, doing. The doing part is one thing but then when someone gives you a bit of encouragement to do it, it works. It's more powerful than the doing on its own. It's like the affirmation or something. If a fella affirms you for doing one thing it's more powerful than doing a thousand things.
>
> (Jack)

For many, being part of a friendly paid or unpaid workforce meant that it was impossible to avoid inclusion, and this reinforced the realization, first experienced in GROW, that 'I am not so different from others'. Kate noted that being at work provided a whole range of social connections, and Penny affirmed the value she placed on a regular unpaid role she had taken on in a day center:

> In an environment like that where you have so many people you can't sit on your own, there are 300 people out for a break at the one time. You get sucked along with the crowd. You go out for a smoke break and there are 20 outside. You can't help but be drawn in.
>
> (Kate)

I love the people there I would not miss going, I've made an awful lot of friends, they come from the town and from the countryside, people I didn't know at all.

(Penny)

By being regularly involved in work (paid or unpaid) and enjoying the company of other people, the hold of traumas from the past, or what Frank (1995) describes as 'bits and pieces of memory that came from another time', began to loosen. Kate, Peter and Jack had all come from positions of hopelessness. Kate 'felt suicide was the only way to get rid of this'; Peter 'would have been happy to give up on life' and Jack said 'I can't go on, everything was just on top of me'; now they began to find a security in work, and a multitude of positive little things began to reassure them that they were on their way to recovery.

Frank suggests that testimonies of wellness present as 'some fragment of a larger whole that the individual witness makes no pretense of grasping in its entirety' (Frank 1995:139). Author C. S. Lewis, in his autobiography *Surprised by Joy* (1955), described how moments of joy acted as beacons of hope that sustained him through dark passages of life. Kate, Jack and Peter and others had entered a time of positive becoming, an ongoing process of which they were only partly aware. Fragments of daily experiences, such as throwing themselves into work, huddling with others over a cigarette, opening a pay packet, experiencing the satisfaction of being trusted, being praised and making friends, all became multiple sources of new memories for participants – memories that created a whole new range of 'proximal processes' (Bronfenbrenner 1977), which further nurtured resilience and recovery. These memories were experienced primarily as hopeful or joyful feelings, somatic stories, a new song in people's hearts, hearts that were no longer just physical pumps but 'hearts that leapt with joy' (Deegan 1995:91) and which confirmed each person as a unique, valid and valued human being.

In this next extract, Kate describes a real sense of having become an independent person. Unlike the hope that first beckoned at the start of her encounter with GROW and which, in some mysterious way, was transferred to her from others, the exhilaration she now felt was the product of her own 're-authoring' or 'story-work'. It was not the end point of her journey but confirmation that she was journeying in the direction to becoming her 'ideological self' and a call for further choices. Kate began to experience a deep excitement about the possibilities life might be able to offer her, another self-generated 'somatic' story that encouraged her to renew her efforts on her journey.

I remember one of my first social nights out, without any of my safety nets like GROW or my husband, was actually in that job. I went out one night for the Christmas break and again that sense of I'm actually out for a night and my husband isn't here, that whole sense of standing on my own two feet was exhilarating to say the least . . . All these things were laying the foundation for me to go on to bigger and better things . . . All of these things were a challenge and every challenge I took on drove me forward a little step. And every challenge I took on maybe made me look at or want to do something else.

(Kate)

Kate had begun to challenge herself, she had 're-authored' her life as a positive unfolding mystery containing opportunities to become. Like Walt Whitman, she could triumphantly sing:

I CELEBRATE myself; houses and rooms are full of perfumes . . . the shelves are crowded with perfumes, I breathe the fragrance myself, and know it and like it. The distillation would intoxicate me also, but I shall not let it. It is for my mouth forever – I am in love with it.

(Whitman 1963:1)

Payment for work is one of the social rituals that educationalist Jerome Bruner (2002:45) says 'frames things in such a way as to be seen as beyond debate'. Many prominent psychiatrists, such as William Anthony (1993) and Arthur Kleinman (Patel and Kleinman 2003), have identified poverty as a significant social determinant of mental health and suggest that ongoing poverty, coupled with low levels of education, mitigate against recovery. Paid employment not only provided a new identity, it provided real resources to cope with 'other forces', such as in Kate's case, where she lived in an area 'notorious for crime and drugs' which threatened her own and her family's well-being. Being in paid employment enabled Kate to choose to move to another area of town:

That job was great for me. It was the first step onto the beginning of a new life. The fact that I returned to work and my husband got work quickly afterwards enabled us to buy our first house. I loved the area I was living in but it became notorious for crime and drugs and it would not have been a nice place to bring my children up in.

(Kate)

For all, paid employment also meant that they now had the resources to become involved in other beneficial social involvements, such as golf (Jack), travelling to football and other sporting events (Peter) or taking a holiday (Mags). Others reported being enabled to access educational courses, such as the leaving certificate (Jess) or a degree programmes in philosophy, science or theology (Helen, David, Cathy).

The healing influence of education

For Jess and for many other participants, the 'distillation' that 'would intoxicate' their lives (Whitman 1963:1) included going back to education. Missing out on the basics of formal education was, for Jess, a huge problem which, through his participation in a weekly support group, he learned to tackle. Once he felt comfortable within the group, Jess found that he could speak about his lack of education, which was a source of stigma and embarrassment, and the group was able to encourage him to access adult education. His first task from the group was to go back to evening classes and complete the junior certificate examination. He was delighted with his own success:

> It was a big thing to tell you the truth, my embarrassment around my lack of education. You know I was [eventually] able to come in and sit in a room and talk about that in front of 10 or 12 people and be able to say, 'I'm out of school since I was 12', something I was even slow to admit to myself, that I didn't have this education. And I knew I was quite capable of it, it wasn't anything beyond me like you know. And I remember getting a challenge from the group to do something about it . . . In the junior cert I did six subjects and I got six As and I was delighted with myself. I did it after work, I used to go off down to the adult education. It took me 2 years. And I tell you now in that side of my life that has been the biggest change was my junior cert.
>
> (Jess)

After the success of the junior certificate examination, Jess went on to successfully complete his leaving certificate examination and began to realize that these achievements were putting him in a position where he could choose to leave his current employment. With the encouragement of the group and his wife, Jess then decided to apply for a course in computers because it was something he found personally interesting. Taking on full-time third-level study proved very challenging and, in Jess's opinion, was only possible because of his experience of being supported to face challenges within the context of the GROW group.

> I have to say now the first day in college was one of the most daunting days I had in my life and if it wasn't for GROW I'd have walked out, because I was standing there, I was the oldest in the class. There was 120 of us going in for this course day one . . . And I was able to stand there, think about stuff, like parts of the GROW program that come into your head like, 'do the ordinary thing you fear, do the ordinary thing that repels you'.
>
> (Jess)

While Jess (and others) described how a return to education removed a sense of stigma and provided a new sense of identity, many participants reported that going back to formal education helped them form a new and meaningful understanding of life which they found to be very empowering, countering the nihilism of terror and the label of 'mental illness'. More than one third of the participants reported various benefits of studying philosophy or theology.

David was already in secure employment, but a course in philosophy helped him make sense of life and relationships:

> I discovered philosophy. Gabriel Marcel, a Christian existentialist. He kind of believes in our relationships with people we create. We're creative in our

relationships with other people, and hence the meaning of harmony in relationships is what it's all about. I became more philosophically aware.

(David)

Similarly, Cathy found that studying theology placed her in the midst of a group
of people with whom she felt profoundly at home. She felt she had been connected to love, and this was, for her, a life changing experience:

It was wonderful to sit in a class. I think I loved it. I did a 3-year course . . . That
whole issue of wanting to get to know what is it all about. So I think I wanted
to know God better. It was very helpful because I got insight into the spirituality side of it. To know how you know. We do things, that's a choice we
took at that particular time. Don't sort of analyse it. Just say well that was a
learning process, like what would I do different the next time? And that was
theology. It was very practical.

(Cathy)

Theology gave Cathy some tools to help her understand herself and made life
more manageable by opening up the possibility that life was composed of choices
and 'I would do [things] different the next time', thus opening a future that held
the promise of 're-authorship'.

Mathew studied theology independently through reading books. He had lived
with a psychiatric identity for many years and wanted to know more about the
reality of 'mental illness' (apart from the crippling medical story), so he began to
search for new explanations that would perhaps allow him to understand himself
in a new way. Different books provided fragments of insight which collectively
offered new ways of understanding all the 'crazy experiences' about which, for
17 years, doctors 'wouldn't tell you much'.

For 17 years. They [the psychiatrists and nurses] wouldn't tell you much.
They might spend a minute or two telling you about whatever it was. It was
on my own bat I actually went out and found out about what 'mental illness'
is, first of all what 'manic depression' was and then what 'schizoaffective'
was. I suppose, all those sort of crazy experiences kind of triggered an interest in spirituality. After the age of 31 or 32 I was reading an awful lot of
spiritual books, I must have read about 80 or 90 spiritual books in the last 8
or 9 years. In a practical way, it's helped me. I saw a common thread between
Christian mystics and Taoism and Zen.

(Mathew)

Just as work stopped Kate thinking about herself, thus providing space for the
'authorisation' of new stories; Mathew found that the practice of meditation
brought the same result.

A lot of it is just slow your thinking down, come out of your head. The real
part of you, the part of you that feels most alive and most spacious. Most of

life is not the fearful little voice in your head, it's the silence, it's the heart or the soul, the spirit down here, it's quiet, it's not thinking, it's not conceptual intelligence, it's just pure consciousness, pure awareness.

(Mathew)

In the study of meditative techniques, Mathew had stumbled on (or been led to) a therapeutic strategy inspired by studies which show that Buddhist meditation techniques are 'useful for patients who have not responded to more traditional forms of psychotherapy' (Whitaker 2010).

The healing influence of leisure-based involvements

While employment and education played key roles in their recovery, many participants described leisure involvements that were also helpful to the process of recovery. For example, golf played an unexpectedly key role in James's recovery. Just as in the early days of James's involvement in GROW, at the golf club, there was a relaxed atmosphere and he immediately felt at home. He soon realised golf had an unexpected agenda that enabled him to understand himself in new ways.

In work they had a golf society. I went along to the first golf outing and everyone there was very courteous and there was no bravado, it was a very relaxed atmosphere. The one thing I noticed about golf was that, my anger levels would build up, you know tension. I could start off okay. Through not being able to hit it, now that's perfectly natural in golf, but for me it was building up to real bad levels of stress. Yeah, so the task was to be aware of it. I also noticed that when the anger would build up also my sense of perception would lose itself. The more my anger built up the more I felt that people were out to get me.

(James)

Gradually, James realised that golf, because it increased his stress levels, triggered his old feelings of anger-filled paranoia. This realisation allowed him to discover new ways of dealing with it. Golf had become a biofeedback mechanism through which he could practice the choice of control:

I realized there was a link there between the two, anger and people being out to get me. So a lot of the tasks that I had were to play golf to relax. It's in all the golf books (laughing), saying it's all about the journey, it's about enjoying it, don't think of the result, so some of the golf books have it.

(James)

Through playing golf, anger had been identified as a 'deterministic force' that could be countered by the simple act of conscious relaxation:

The golf definitely helped me in terms of understanding my temperament without a doubt. Now I play with different people every week, just put my name down and some people are very relaxed, and some people will get the clubs and throw them into hedges. And I can look at that person and go well that was me a year ago you know [laughing].

(James)

James's temperament was becoming understandable and manageable. He realized that anger could make other people behave in irrational ways, it wasn't just something that happened to him. This realisation allowed him to 're-author his story'. Instead of seeing himself as some kind of alien, he realized he was pretty much the same as everyone else. He also realized that he had learned how to control his feelings of anger and could trust himself to be at home with others.

Other people in this study reported choosing to become involved in a range of leisure activities, such as creative writing, public speaking, dancing, music, cycling, singing, hill walking, their church, yoga, football and theatre, all of which became micro schools of experiential learning. Like GROW, these groups readily welcomed new members and created other context for new dialogues and tales of relationships of mutuality, belonging, trust and possibility, all of which become part of the person's story of recovery.

A number of participants explicitly stated that social involvements outside GROW were essential to their recovery process. For example, Cathy and Peter described their experience in the following quotations:

You are sent out . . . Whether it's personal development or dance classes . . . wherever a person needs to go . . . I don't think somebody in GROW can 'become', if you keep together . . . you're sent out to build up your own social network, so you don't become isolated within GROW and stigmatised again, that would cause people to be stunted nearly.

(Cathy)

For the recovery model to work well you need different things. I compare it to a stool. If a stool has one or two legs it's unstable but if it has three or four it becomes really stable. For me having GROW was good but having work and things like hill walking helped too.

(Peter)

Concluding comments

Social inclusion, involvement and integration into mainstream community life have long been recognised as essential to the maintenance of mental health and key ingredients of recovery (Huxley and Thornicroft 2001, Department of Health and Children 2006, Cobigo and Stuart 2010). As people continued their recovery they described the positive effects of choosing to become involved in society through paid and unpaid work, through education or through involvements in leisure-based organizations. During their time in GROW, people had been systematically encouraged to take on a range of responsibilities, to make choices and to take personal risks as they learned recovery skills. Now they were actively supported by other GROW members to risk leaving the sheltered environment of peer support and enter a wider social context. GROW had empowered participants to 'gather' qualities such as courage (Kate), resolve (Jess) and strength (Claire) that now enabled them to succeed in a much less supportive and larger social world. Indeed, people were of the view that not to become involved outside the supportive environment of GROW could lead to another form of isolation and stigmatisation.

Social involvement in work, education and leisure provided people with opportunities to adopt a range of new identities associated with being an employee, student or member of a leisure organization. Both education and employment also provided people with access to very real financial and educational resources that increased their ability to choose the next step in their chosen life path. Participants' accounts clearly suggested that relationships within these chosen social niches, where people were 'the same as myself', helped eradicate any lingering sense of stigma, shame or sense of being 'other'.

References

Anthony, W. A. 1993. Recovery from mental illness: The guiding vision of the mental health service system in the 1990s. *Psychosocial Rehabilitation Journal*, 16, 521–537.

Bronfenbrenner, U. 1977. Toward an experimental ecology of human development. *American Psychologist*, 32, 513.

Bruner, J. 2002. *Making stories: Law, literature, life*, Cambridge, MA, London, Harvard University Press.

Cobigo, V. & Stuart, H. 2010. Social inclusion and mental health. *Current Opinion in Psychiatry*, 23, 453–457.

Deegan, P. 1995. Coping with recovery as a journey of the heart. *Psychiatric Rehabilitation Journal*, 19, 91–97.

Department of Health and Children 2006. *A vision for change: Report of the expert group on mental health policy*, Dublin, Stationery Office.

Frank, A. 1995. *The wounded storyteller: Body, illness, and ethics*, Chicago, University of Chicago Press.

Huxley, P. & Thornicroft, G. 2001. Social inclusion, social quality and mental illness. *The British Journal of Psychiatry*, 182, 289–290.

Lewis, C. S. 1955. *Surprised by Joy: The shape of my early life*, New York, Harcourt Books.

Patel, V. & Kleinman, A. 2003. Poverty and common mental disorders in developing countries. *Bulletin of the World Health Organization*, 81, 609–615.

Whitaker, R. 2010. *Anatomy of an epidemic: Magic bullets, psychiatric drugs, and the astonishing rise of mental illness in America*, New York, Random House.

Whitman, W. 1963. *Leaves of grass*, London, Penguin.

12 Flourishing selves and a re-enchantment with life

I'm going to Lourdes in September, I might be going to Malta for Christmas with my girlfriend and that will be all for this year. If we do that it will create another record. I have records being broken all the time you know. The crowning glory was a trip to China and I was in Egypt and to think all that, I would have loved to have done that years ago but I didn't have the confidence.

(Pat)

You know, it's amazing now that I can just go over [to neighbours I used to avoid], I can go into town, I can go to Church and do the ordinary things . . . I did a few interviews on radio and all that helped. I began to believe in myself . . . I began to believe well, look Nan 'you are as good as anyone, as the next person'. I stopped all the criticising of myself and exchanged them [negative comments] for positive comments.

(Nan)

Successful involvement in society is often seen as the main destination or the end point of recovery. For the 26 people whose stories made up this narrative, successful social involvement was clearly not the end of recovery, but represented an exciting new beginning. For them, recovery appeared to be a never-ending process of discovery. Through their apprenticeship within GROW people had commenced their recovery journey and developed a genuine sense of possibility, including the ability to imagine realistic options for the future. Through others' help and ongoing nurturing, they eventually developed the confidence and ability to access the worlds of education, employment and leisure. Through this involvement, they began to flourish as capable human beings and developed a deep knowledge of themselves and their potential. They were also developing a realistic sense of their own durability and what they needed to do to stay on the recovery journey and remain mentally well. Although they were aware that their mental health was not to be taken for granted, this awareness was not something that gave rise to fear but an embodied sense that their vulnerability was now a strength to be used for the benefit of others. As they flourished people reported tackling life problems and situations that in the past had disempowered them. They also reported a strong desire to give back to society, to reach out to others and to contribute their wisdom to the social good.

Understanding my recovery and what it means for me

As people successfully navigated their way into society, through involvement in education, work and leisure, they began to experience an exhilarating sense of a range of possibilities that lay ahead. It was as if all the painstaking work accomplished since joining peer support was suddenly bearing fruit. They began to blossom and to experience a real zest for life, looking forward to their future. At this stage, participants were also demonstrating a real depth of self-knowledge and understanding of their own life situation, so that each person's flourishing became uniquely personal. For each, finding the next step was about understanding their unique life situation in order to map out and experiment with ways of being, behaving and living that enabled them to grow and mature into the future. Participants provided numerous examples of how they were now empowered to tackle particular social situations that in the past had contributed to their sense of powerlessness and inability to cope with life.

Cathy, for example, described how some of her distress had been precipitated by participation in a committee that was full of conflict. Flourishing, in her situation, meant learning how to successfully deal with similar sources of conflict. In GROW and later in work, she learned how to successfully absorb tension and discomfort without feeling overwhelmed and was no longer threatened by people who held views that differed from her own.

> I suppose for me it was learning maturity as an adult. That I didn't always have to agree, and it was okay to disagree. Even now being able to express something, whether somebody likes it or not. A big step forward for me was learning to express it [own view], and that it's okay to disagree. Agree to disagree and not avoid.
>
> (Cathy)

For Peter, a key part of his recovery lay in learning how to make friends and work cooperatively with others. He discovered, first, through participation in GROW that he could learn to control his anger, which always lurked beneath the surface, especially when he perceived other people to be 'difficult'. For many years Peter had avoided all friendly contact with people, including members of his own family. Peter talked about how he discovered that changing his attitude and behaviour, by being friendly with, respectful of and cooperative towards others radically changed his relationships in a way that was personally liberating and which allowed him to flourish.

> I developed the ability to form friendships and learned how to deal with people even when they were very difficult. I learned to keep my negative feelings under control. You know it's very easy to be kind of negative and critical of other people, but the whole issue of understanding and seeing the good in others, and maybe accepting that they have a dark side too, forced me to learn skills I wouldn't normally have been disciplined enough to learn, I mean communication and emotion.
>
> (Peter)

Richard slowly learned to accept and deal with the pain of an unwanted and devastating marriage separation. Again, a combination of support from members of the group and a process of personal change, wrought through his involvement within GROW, formed Richard's apprenticeship to learning to deal with life. To illuminate the change and learning, Richard compared the deep sense of guilt and self-blame he experienced at the time of his marriage breakdown to his present perspective:

> One of the guys that was there when I joined said 'Richard, you were scary to look at', he says, 'the lights were on, but there was nobody home!'. And I remember, when it come round to my turn, I'd try to speak, I'd try to say something, and I'd just start crying. I could see people, you know, they were taking one problem, and they were working on that, they could make progress with one thing at a time. And this was great, rather than being overwhelmed by everything. Eventually I found that my own mountains slowly became [re-framed as] molehills and life became manageable. But I have to say, with the benefit of hindsight, for me personally, if you could take the kids out of it, she [my wife] did me a tremendous service by ending the marriage, I wouldn't be able to put up with her nowadays, not at all. I'm a very different person now, you know.
>
> (Richard)

Nan's unique journey of self-understanding and management centered around learning how to believe in herself, learning to choose to be happy and live in the here and now:

> I began to believe in myself, that's all I can say. My philosophy would be to get up in the morning, be as happy as you can, do the best you can. Another technique that helped me was living in the now. Enjoying the moment, just this moment. You will never have it again, just live in the moment.
>
> (Nan)

In Nan's view, evidence of her flourishing came through her increasing ability to enjoy the little things in life and an emerging confidence which had begun to replace the once-familiar emotional 'story' of fear, which had followed her since her early childhood:

> With time I did begin to feel good about myself and I actually learned to love myself which was a great thing. It's the small things in life that keep me happy, it's the small things, nothing big, you know smelling a rose for instance is a lovely thing, sitting out in the garden and having a cup of coffee, the small things . . . The confidence you gain in GROW no one can ever take that away from you. It's there for life and it's wonderful to feel good about yourself. I think GROW is a testing ground, it helped me enormously with my own personal life.
>
> (Nan)

Helen too described how a combination of GROW, work and social involvements gave her a deep sense of unexpected happiness.

> Well happiness, happiness is a good experience and you know, you're feeling better, your face is brighter and your eyes are sparkling and your smiling and you're not worried and life is good. I'd be driving over some days to work and I said, oh I'm so happy, you know, this is a great experience. I never thought after a difficult life [I had] I'd get a break at forty-six, and find myself working at something and being happy. I'm going to enjoy it while I have it: the social side and the work side and the achievement and the structure to my days, of the week, and the income, I think the social contact and the kindness of people.
>
> (Helen)

Many participants reported that an important part of their recovery and emotional development involved learning to embrace and find meaning in different forms of suffering rather than running away from them. This was very evident in Nan's account. Nan has a daughter, Leah, with a severe neurological condition for whom she is a full-time carer. For Nan, recovering and flourishing involved accepting this situation which contained truly awful memories of Leah's physical distress. While still challenging for both Nan and Leah, today Nan has 're-framed' the way she sees Leah's life and her purpose in life. She describes it as almost a blessing which has given her daughter's life a marvellous purpose.

> People come up to me and Leah, it's like a magic energy in her. You'd see it if you meet her, she touches off people. And I think Leah is a reason, people have said to me, they might be going on about something, someone sick, and then they might say sure look at Leah you know she, she's no speech or anything and yet she's so happy, so happy. It's remarkable, she touches people.
>
> (Nan)

Giving back: Transforming suffering into the social good

The theme of goodness has been a recurrent feature of different people's recovery stories. Recovery involved an ethical transformation with a continued emphasis on choosing to 'do the good and ordinary thing . . . the thing you fear . . . the thing that repelled you' rather than doing what your feelings might suggest, such as a withdrawal from others and from life (GROW 2001:3). As people began to resolve past suffering and hurts and became increasingly involved in society, they overwhelmingly reported a desire to give back to others.

Kate, who initially returned to the workforce as an assembly-line worker, eventually went on to train as a psychotherapist. During that programme she soon realised that her past suffering and her journey to recovery were resources that in some way set her positively (rather than negatively) apart from others on the course.

> I wanted to recover, I wanted to learn, I wanted to change my life and become. Exactly just become, and my suffering taught me to do that, and it was invaluable

when it came to talking about yourself. What I had learned in GROW was like manna from heaven. They [the others on the course] were so [emotionally] removed from themselves. When it came then the real crunch in that kind of training, if your own house isn't sorted out, you cannot sit with another person's pain, you just can't. It [suffering] is the thing that can teach us the lessons.

(Kate)

Kate's suffering had become meaningful as she began to change. Now, as she looked back on her own recovery journey, she could see how these experiences were of immense value to others. Similarly, until she had experienced a mental health problem herself, Martha could never understand why a young woman that she worked with could be depressed. She felt her own experience made her a better and more empathetic person, a person that could now reach out to and be more supportive of people in similar situations.

Yeah, it [experiencing a mental health problem] makes you a better person, it changes your way of thinking, before I got sick I would have, like okay maybe there'd be some girls inside [work] and there'd be days they wouldn't be well and I'd say god what's wrong with them, 19-, 20-year-olds, what the hell are they playing at, I wouldn't really have the understanding anything like the understanding I would have now. Before I got sick, depression was something you kind of, you got yourself up in a heap over nothing, I could never understand somebody, take a young girl, 20 years of age, she had her job, she had her boyfriend, everything was going grand for [her]. So it [experiencing a mental health problem] would have given me a huge understanding for people's pain and suffering, GROW completely changed my outlook on life.

(Martha)

As Claire recovered from the grief of losing her grandson and then her son to suicide, she came to a point where she decided she should use her own suffering to reach out to others. Claire's devastating loss was no longer the end but became the beginning of social outreach work. What Frank (1992:467) has termed 'the pedagogy of suffering', a pedagogy that transforms suffering into a deeply understood compassion for others, came calling across the airwaves when Claire heard another lady's story on the radio. Claire recalls:

It [GROW] made me that strong that after about 2 years I thought, 'What can I do about this now to help prevent suicide?' I got it into my mind I'd like to bring something to this part of Ireland and I heard a lady on the radio one day. She lost her son, a 16-year-old, and she started a youth suicide campaign. So I got in touch with her and I thought it was going to happen tomorrow, I had no idea the work that does go on, but anyway we got there after about 2 years, loads of fundraising events and things like that and we now have three phone lines operating in [names town].

(Claire)

Whilst GROW had given Claire the strength to contribute to the social good in a bigger way, she soon learned that setting up a helpline was a journey that required huge effort that unfolded over a long period of time. As she told her story on local radio, a community began to grow around her. Claire was soon identified by others as a woman of strength and compassion, someone who had suffered and someone who understood their suffering and fears. By publicly telling her story she set in motion a dialogue about the modern-day epidemic of suicide among young Irish men, which many people had struggled to engage with. Claire became the yeast of change. Everyone knew someone who had died by suicide, everyone was affected by the unfolding story.

Pat, who had been afraid even to leave his own home for a number of years, even to buy food, described how he became involved in his local parish as a way of giving back and that this confirmed, for him, the reality of his recovery:

I actually began to feel a bit well out on the street, this is the way it went off and then I got involved in the committee up in the local parish centre . . . I really blossomed.

(Pat)

Without exception all the participants in this study reported a desire to use their own unique experience of suffering as a reason to give back, both as leaders in GROW and through wider community and social involvements. Paul, for whom opportunities for giving back were severely restricted because he was in various prisons or secure units, reported becoming sacristan in the secure unit's small church and took on a leadership role within GROW within the unit. Several participants gave back by becoming full-time area coordinators within GROW, two became regional chair people, one was employed as manager of a women's refuge and another became involved in working with the deaf community. Tom's recovery began with attempts to become involved in small informal social events. At one such event he met a girl who was deaf with whom he felt very much at ease. Seeing people using sign language struck him as an interesting alternative way to communicate and led to his long-term involvement with the deaf community.

As I grew a wee bit more in confidence I got involved, I met a deaf girl, who I was very friendly with for a while. And then I met another friend of hers, who is deaf, but her speech you could just about make it out, but she couldn't lip read. So one deaf girl would sort of interpret to the other. And I seen the sign language, and I thought 'that's a fascinating language here'. So she introduced me to the Deaf Fellowship in [mentions name of town] she said 'they're an older group, and they'll tolerate someone like you with some learning'. So I went to class here to learn basic sign language.

(Tom)

Unaccountable aspects of recovery: Providence or chance

Whilst each person described their story of recovery in a fairly logical and sequential manner, most of these stories also contained accounts of mysterious coincidences which many described as providential or chance events. Whilst they were both timely and helpful, they went beyond logical explanations. This idea that 'chance events' reflect a greater order and meaning in life than we are normally aware of is reflected in Jung's concept of synchronicity (Jung 1965). Jung believed that life is not a series of random events but rather an expression of a deeper order '*Unus mundus*'. Jung based this belief on experiences within his own life and within therapy. A female client was relating a dream which featured a golden scarab beetle. As she spoke a real scarab beetle began to tap at the window. The scarab in Egyptian mythology represents rebirth. From a religious perspective Jung (1965) believed that synchronicity served a similar role in a person's life to dreams, with the purpose being to shift a person's egocentric conscious thinking to greater wholeness. From the religious perspective synchronicity shares similar characteristics of an 'intervention of grace'. It is not dissimilar to the Buddhist notion of karma or the Christian idea of trusting in the munificence of a loving God. In Lundstrom's (1996:176) view synchronicity is 'a glimpse into an underlying order in the universe, which manifests itself through meaningful coincidences that cannot be explained by cause and effect'.

Peg's recovery narrative included many unexplainable and seemingly chance 'co-incidences', such as finding work at a time of great need and obtaining a mortgage through a chance meeting with a car park attendant who used to work in a bank:

> I would say things happen to me that are beyond explaining except as part of providence.

(Peg)

Kate, similarly, found shift work that coincided with her growing family's needs.

> The job was almost like divine intervention, the hours just suited and matched my husband's.

(Kate)

Frances saw it as being providential that, with no direct plan on her part and having lived all over the world, she found herself living and working in the area where she had grown up as a foster child. As a foster child, living in that place, her life had been dominated by feelings of rejection and alienation. Now she felt she had come full circle and, having integrated her past in a way that was no longer painful or shameful, she was very much at home and glad to be back there, as she now had a strong sense of personal identity and was happy with who she was.

> Providence features greatly in my life. I have come full circle and ended up a few miles from where I was brought up. I no longer need to avoid my neighbours.
>
> (Frances)

Pat understood providence as being linked to his own behaviour and willingness to change. As he cooperated with different kinds of help from others, he developed a feeling that he was being providentially led, as he said 'being ready and providence are linked' (Pat). Tom, in a similar vein, associated providence with his attempts to become increasingly involved in society and was of the view that it was only when you open yourself up to involvements with other people that providence had a chance to intervene.

> If you only get involved in something small you meet people that lead to the next one [involvement] and so forth and so the net widens.
>
> (Tom)

James was feeling very exposed and vulnerable after his story of mental distress and recovery had appeared in a national newspaper. As he began to question his decision about completing the interview for the paper, he was reassured on his way to work by a chance encounter with a colleague who had read the interview.

> It was amazing that he (a friendly work colleague) just happened to be coming out at that time and he told me that I did the right thing.
>
> (James)

Frances and Mags both reported hearing personal testimonies at their first meeting of GROW that appeared to be tailor made to their own particular needs. Could this have been an example of synchronicity or providentiality? What are the odds of a particular storyteller being in a GROW meeting on the very night that Frances or Mags came?

While many participants actively promoted the idea of the existence of providence, David dismissed the idea.

> I would be nervous of interpreting things like providence, it could be madness again, if I start attributing significance to incidents that happened I know I am going in the wrong direction.
>
> (David)

Concluding comments

This, the final chapter about people's recovery journeys, views recovery as a continuous process of discovery, which leads to a flourishing self and 'a re-enchantment with life'. Flourishing involves learning how to resolve past suffering, learning how to enjoy the present, and choosing a life path that enables each person to blossom. Participants indicated that recovery from mental distress transformed them from being passively dependent on the help of others to being an invaluable and generous resource for other people. As a consequence, 'a re-enchantment with life' also included a growing desire to reach out to others, with many people describing how they had found ways to contribute to the social good by becoming involved in outreach projects.

The possible existence of a benign providence was a common belief among many participants. Many people offered examples of how they had been significantly helped in very practical yet mysterious ways in their journey from despair to hope, from sadness to joy and from alienated isolation to rewarding meaningful life and involvement within society.

References

Frank, A. W. 1992. The pedagogy of suffering moral dimensions of psychological therapy and research with the ill. *Theory & Psychology*, 2, 467–485.

GROW 2001. *Program of growth to maturity*, Sydney, GROW Publications.

Jung, C. G. 1965. *Memories, dreams, reflections*, New York, Random House.

Lundstrom, M. 1996. What is synchronicity? 'A wink from the cosmos'. *Intuition Magazine* (May), 176–180.

13 Recovery through mutual help

Recovery processes revisited

> Practicing in different worlds, groups of scientists see different things when they look from the same point in the same direction. Again, that is not to say that they can see anything they please. Both are looking at the world, and what they look at has not changed. But in some areas they see different things, and they see them in different relations one to another.
>
> (Kuhn 1962:149)

The cumulative narratives of the 26 people whose stories inform this study have been woven by us into a 'second-order narrative', which Elliott (2005:10) suggests is 'the account a researcher constructs to make sense of the social world and of other people's experiences'. By exploring mental distress through a narrative methodology, as opposed to using a more traditional research methodology, we were enabled as Kuhn (1962:149) suggests to see different things and different relationships.

These narratives suggest that recovery, like life, is an ongoing, non-linear journey, but also like life, is one with recognisable developmental processes or stages. As an outcome of developing a second-order narrative, recovery was presented in the previous chapters as a process of ongoing personal transformation conceptualised as 'a re-enchantment with life'.

'Re-enchantment' began when people escaped from 'places of terror' by joining the mutual-support group of GROW. Here they received a warm and emotional welcome which they described as an enchanting encounter with hope. Hopeful feelings gave rise to unexpectedly hopeful ways of thinking which in turn re-directed people towards a healing community and away from isolation. 'Re-enchantment' was systematically nurtured through 'a time of healing' within the social womb of GROW. The GROW group became a place where people tried out different life strategies and learned from experience, becoming experts in what worked for them. Over time the regular witnessing of their own and others' efforts at recovery began to build resilience, which eventually enabled people to reconnect with others outside of GROW and within niches in society. Society now represented 'an opportunity to become', and offered a range of meaningful involvements which enabled ongoing development and growth and where each person began to flourish with an evident zest for living and a desire to help others.

As an outcome of the analysis, a number of nurturing or recovery processes have been identified, which we believe work in harmony to enable each person's recovery path to unfold naturally, within the context of their emerging capabilities. We have named these nurturing processes as experiencing empathic and compassionate witness, becoming hopeful and believing in possibility, reconnecting with self and others, participating in positive and helpful risk taking, re-authoring a more positive identity, being the helper as well as the helped, transforming understanding of self and distress and engaging with the spiritual dimension of self.

The focus of this chapter is on discussing and theorising how these nurturing or enabling recovery processes merged together in a manner that acknowledged the uniqueness of each person's story and allowed each person to travel their own journey, at their own pace, whilst ensuring that mutual support was a constant presence to scaffold and support.

Experiencing empathic and compassionate witness

A consistent feature of each person's story was the absence of a compassionate other to whom they could relate their pain and who could thereby bring some relief. Hence, the most important starting point of each person's recovery was the act of bearing witness. Bearing witness, in the context of mutual support, was about 'being with', 'engaging with' and 'caring with' each other in an empathic and compassionate manner. It initially consisted of listening to and bearing witness to other people's stories while slowly allowing others to bear witness to one's own story of distress and pain. According to Charon (2006:65), 'telling of pain and suffering [and] giving voice to what they [people] endure' is critical to any healing process. Frank (2002:123) suggests that people need 'to witness their own suffering and to express this experience so that the rest of us can learn from it'. Bearing witness through storytelling served a number of functions.

Within the 'carnival atmosphere' (Bakhtin 1981) of peer support, a context where 'matters pertaining to diagnosis and treatment and technical language from psychiatry are banned' (GROW 2001:20), people were able to experience themselves not as patients, clients or some kind of alien 'other' set apart from 'normality' but as people struggling together with various problems of living and with a mysteriously unfolding life. To discover that other people faced similar kinds of struggles and distress not only normalised feelings of isolation, but validated people's experiences of trauma, as their distress was witnessed, believed and heard, often for the first time. This profound realisation of sameness cut away a deep-rooted sense of otherness and a wish to be left alone.

Listening to other people's stories also provided very practical information about the process of recovery. It broke down the journey into different phases or stages, providing information on how people began, information on who and what helped along the way, information on what happened in times of setbacks, plus it gave people an understanding of what people hoped for in the future. By listening to the stories of others, people realised that recovery takes time and involves taking ownership and a willingness to take small risks.

People described experiencing storytelling within the group as a homecoming; it created a place where they belonged, connected and felt profoundly at home. Central to these feelings of belonging and connectedness was the ability of people within the group to suspend what Rowan and Jacobs (2002:76) described as 'the separateness of the self' and enter the heart, mind and world of the other person. It was in these 'I–Thou' moments that the process of collaborative healing took place. People's narratives indicated that bearing witness to each person's efforts, durability, courage and resourcefulness was equally important as witnessing their distress and woundedness. Thus, an interpersonal milieu of healing was created that not only acted as a powerful source of hope for people, but it enhanced people's sense of control and power, leading to increased confidence and trust in one's abilities, resourcefulness and voice. People were inspired to continue their recovery journey in the knowledge that the group was a safe place to risk new thoughts and actions and would always be there to offer encouragement.

Becoming hopeful and believing in possibility

Hope is increasingly recognised by service users (Chamberlin 1978, Deegan 1995, Coleman 2004, Fisher 2005) and mental health professionals (Maddock and Hallam 2010, Leamy *et al.* 2011) as an important element of people's recovery. Deegan (1995), one of the key leaders in the mental health service user movement, claims that 'hope is not just a nice sounding euphemism [but] is a matter of life or death' (Deegan 1995:3). Yet despite its centrality to recovery, Stuart (2010:361) believes it is 'the most absent, ingredient in contemporary mental health care'. People's narratives provide some understanding of how hope 'works', suggesting that it is something that can be appropriated or transferred from one person to another and communicated to people through powerful but often non-verbal forms of language.

Frank (1995) suggests that as the body speaks at a depth that is initially beyond understanding, consequently it takes time for each individual to construct a meaning and plan a course of action in response to bodily feelings. Hope was first experienced as a sensation or existential feeling registered deep inside the physical body and was described in the first instance as a 'promising somatic story'. It was triggered by experiencing a warm and emotional welcome from friendly peers. These initial sensations of hope brought about a sense of tranquillity at a somatic level, which was closely linked to the awakening of other positive emotional states, such as joy, acceptance, warmth and belonging. For all participants, this unexpected and powerful somatic or body story was a critical point in their journey, as it gave each person permission to allow the emergence of new and exciting thoughts about themselves and their future. Though at first these positive thoughts and emotions were very fragile and embryonic, the possibility of things being better, even though the person did not fully understand how this might happen, acted as an internal prompt to return to the group week after week.

Within the group, hope was nurtured by the experience of genuinely reciprocal care by others. What was first experienced as a 'possibility of hope' slowly opened the way for the emergence of new ways of being and interacting with the world. Gradually, seminal ideas from GROW became part of each person's world-view, so that thoughts such as 'I can and will recover' or 'No-one is a no hoper' (GROW 2001:50) replaced the pessimistic professional and cultural stories of 'mental illness', which had previously dominated people's thinking. Through the ongoing application of GROW's transformative principles, people soon learned to have a genuine sense of what might be possible in the future and apply the maxims to 'do the good and ordinary thing you fear' and to 'think by reason rather than by feelings and imagination' (GROW 2001:5–7).

People's hopeful beliefs were justified and continually nurtured by witnessing and hearing the testimony of other people in the group who were further along the road of recovery. Other group members acted as beacons of hope and role models, providing inspiration, strengthening people's resolve and helping them mobilize their energy to move forward. Cheered on and inspired by others, each person systematically and gradually gathered resources, such as courage, wisdom and endurance. Through immersion in reciprocal relationships where people shared leadership and friendship, people grew in hope and began to realise their own power and grasped the exciting idea that they were as valuable as anyone else. With this realisation and the ongoing support of others, people began to realis-tically believe and work towards a positive future. They identified and strove to accomplish manageable goals appropriate to their unique stage of recovery, despite limitations and ongoing challenges. As they progressed from an 'appren-ticeship in peer support', they successfully took their place in society, where they became 'holders of hope' for others who needed support.

Re-connecting with self and others

People react to trauma in very unique and individual ways, depending on the nature of the trauma, how they appraise the event, presence or absence of coping strategies, reactions of others including family and the wider community and the availability of supportive others (Lanius *et al.* 2010). When people experience trauma their whole world is disrupted and their assumptions of a just and caring world are challenged (Frank 1995). At the same time instincts of self-preservation are heightened, and people withdraw as a means of self-protection, either through choice or as a result of the absence of a caring other. Whilst withdrawal can be a useful short-term strategy, in the long term it leaves people isolated and impris-oned by their distressing thoughts and emotions, which ultimately get labelled as 'mental illness'. Once labelled, a second cycle of exclusion, discrimination and loss of voice is often experienced, tending to propel people into further disconnec-tion, despair and isolation (Thornicroft 2006).

Within this study, in a reverse type of process, people's recovery narratives identified the importance of rebuilding connection with self and others as key to recovery. Participants described how being involved in peer support empow-ered them to move from a time of chaos (Frank 1995), characterised by a loss of connection with self and others, into biographical time (Bakhtin 1981), which involved a reconnection with their own resources and with the compassionate, friendly support of other people.

As people listened to others' stories and recounted and shared their own stories, there was a process of reconnecting with what Browne (2008) refers to as the 'frozen present', feelings and emotions that are suppressed, denied or hidden. Through recounting painful and traumatic experiences with supportive and empathetic others, people began to experience emotional relief, which in turn created space for more creative thinking about the relationship between feelings, thoughts and actions. The warmth of friendly reciprocal interaction within the group generated a range of recovery resources, including: empathy, understanding, acceptance, compassion and love. These resources enabled each person to being the process of whittling away at the walls of fear, mistrust and disconnection and began the process of learning how to compassionately value themselves.

Gradually, through a combination of encouragement and support, each person was challenged to explore the connection between powerful feelings and ways of thinking and behaving. During this time participants learned which of their feelings were worth cultivating and which needed to be intelligently pruned, changed or nurtured. In a cyclical process, as people realised that constructive connections between emotion, thoughts and behaviour could bring about positive personal change, tangible feelings of control, self-efficacy and empowerment increased.

As people began to learn to reconnect with themselves and others within the sheltered 'womb' of the mutual-support group, they were encouraged to reconnect with a wide range of people outside that group. At first these connections were within the larger community of GROW, but increasingly they involved connecting with people in the wider community. People were steered towards different individuals and agencies that might help them continue their journey of recovery and growth. At this point the group could be likened to a beehive and the group members to bees. Each bee was sent out to discover and connect with resources within the community and return to the hive, where they reported on the source, availability and type of support received. In this way, people were being connected to the whole of society and the barriers of stigma and discrimination associated with the label of mental illness were being dismantled.

Participating in positive and helpful risk taking

Research suggests that the dominant risk discourse within mental health services frames risk in negative terms, viewing service users as 'risk-laden objects', with a failure to adopt a positive approach to risk and acknowledge that no action is entirely free of risk (Morgan 2007, Slade 2009, Clancy *et al.* 2014, Higgins *et al.* 2015). Slade (2009:177–178) is of the view that the goal of reducing all risks 'is both damaging and an illusion, . . . [and] can be unintentionally counterproductive, by reducing . . . the extent to which people develop skills at taking responsibility for their own actions'.

Unlike the formal mental health services, which are seen as increasingly trying to tame 'ontological uncertainty' (Rose 1998) through the use of objectifying strategies, including use of risk-prediction assessment tools, and ranking of people within risk categories, mutual support drew heavily on the principle of 'dignity of risk' (Wehmeyer 1998) or GROW's own principle of 'sufficient care, sufficient risk' (GROW 2001:52). Risk was seen as a necessary part of growth and development and something to be embraced as an opportunity. People were not thought of as 'risk objects' but were challenged incrementally to follow their choices, dreams and life goals, even if those choices carried the possibility of failure. By listening to each other's experiences, dreams and wishes, group members supported each other to believe they had the necessary resources and skills to overcome life's challenges in a progressive and systematic way. Instead of being controlled or doubted, each person was trusted to manage themselves and respected to find their own way, with the knowledge that the group was there to support and scaffold them in their endeavours.

By consistently choosing to take small, legitimate risks, people learned how to handle the resultant feelings of stress and fear. People described the steady emergence of resilience and coming to a point where they no longer relied primarily on the support and challenge of others but began to believe that 'I can and even want to do this'. The result of these 'gatherings' of resources over time enabled each person to embrace the challenges and risks involved in entering the world of recreation, education and work.

Within the peer context, effort made was regarded as more important than the immediate results, and setbacks were not viewed as failures and an indication of an inability to make life choices and manage one's life, but were seen as another opportunity for each person to learn. People provided examples where they failed to achieve goals or experienced setbacks but had come to re-frame these as opportunities of self-learning and quoted the GROW maxims 'If a thing is worth doing its worth doing badly for a start, while I am improving' (GROW 2001:32) and 'resume quickly and without fuss' (GROW 2001:15). Setbacks were also opportunities for others to support, provide positive affirmation and celebrate effort. Indeed, at times of setback, people reported being connected to a wealth of positive resources supplied by other members of the group.

Being the helper as well as the helped

The experience of having mental health problems, in itself, is sufficient to engender feelings of uselessness, helplessness and being a burden on others (Amering and Schmolke 2009, Kartalova-O'Doherty *et al.* 2012). This, coupled with the fact that the majority of mental health services people encountered were constructed in a hierarchical manner, which paradoxically reinforced their feelings of helplessness, alienation and disempowerment. The power differential between those delivering a service and those in receipt of a service created a vicious cycle whereby the more professional help the person receives, the greater erosion of their self-efficacy and self-belief and the more dependent they become on others (Loat 2011). The clear delineation made between helper and helped also lead people to believe that they have no value and nothing to offer others (Kloos 1999).

While 'the helper principle' was formally introduced to psychology in 1965 by Riessman, a common theme throughout people's narratives of recovery within this study was the importance of giving back and using their own personal experience of suffering and recovery to help others. Being able to give back was central to the development of people's self-efficacy and feeling of competence. Whilst in the initial phase, people were the recipients of help, support and unconditional acceptance, this quickly developed into a reciprocal process that involved befriending others and supporting them within the group. There was a celebratory connection with personal value, as people discovered that their own pain and their own healing efforts were of value to others in the group.

As people's leadership skills and confidence developed, they moved beyond the safety and comfort of the group and extended help and compassion to sometimes 'unknown' others outside of the group. Whilst all the participants mentioned the importance of re-authoring and developing an identity beyond that of being a 'mentally ill' person, this was not about 'erasing' or hiding that part of their identity but about integrating and reframing their experience of distress, stigma and recovery as an asset as opposed to a liability and using their new-found asset and strength for the benefit of others. For example, Claire established a help line for suicidal teens, Kate became a psychotherapist and Mags became the manager of a hostel for women who had experienced violence.

Re-authoring a more positive identity

As discussed, the label of 'mental illness' often imprisons a person within a negative and toxic identity from which it is difficult to escape (Rappaport 2000), some such identities being that 'I am worthless', 'I am my mental illness' or 'I have no power to change'. These negative scripts arise from dominant cultural narratives about 'mental illness' and those labelled 'mentally ill' and from an internalised sense of stigma. Consequently, there is a widening consensus that developing an alternative positive identity is a key ingredient of recovery (Corrigan *et al.* 2005, Davidson *et al.* 2007, Finn *et al.* 2009).

People's narratives suggest that the process of discovering new and positive identities first began through supportive interactions with others. Sue, who was convinced others would find her unlikable, began to change her view of herself in response to the loving behaviour of another member who proclaimed her to be 'my lovely Sue'. Frances's whole life had been undermined by a series of negative identities, all of which originated from the fact that she had been born illegitimate. She described the powerfully liberating effects of witnessing another person's testimony around being adopted and being valued by the group. Claire found a positive identity through being able to care for a new member, who became 'the son I had lost'.

GROW's inclusive approach to leadership and practical tasks also contributed to identity transformation. Many people mentioned the powerful effect that 'becoming' leaders had on their self-esteem. Taking on roles, such as organiser, implied a belief by others in a person's ability to be responsible. While taking on new roles within the group was initially challenging, over time these acts of leadership enhanced people's belief and trust in themselves and resulted in a re-authored script that now included words of 'ability', 'competence' and 'achievement'. In a cyclical process, each act of leadership within the group enhanced people's willingness to take on additional challenges within and outside the group.

Successful emergence into employment, education, leisure or voluntary work confirmed people's new identities and provided opportunities for other identities to emerge. Being an employee not only provided a concrete social identity but also financial resources which could be used to further tackle the challenges of recovery. Other rewards came in the form of academic qualifications, a release from the stigma attached to low levels of education or being made welcome as fully fledged members of a range of social groups. All of these acted as rites of passage or, as Bruner (2002) describes them, 'social rituals' that changed people's social identities, confirming once again their lack of difference and providing new, challenging contexts for future growth.

Transforming perspectives and understandings of self and distress

Cain (1991), Kennedy (1995), Rappaport (2000) and Rogers and Stanford (2015) all testify that prolonged immersion in a powerful community narrative can bring about a number of important and positive changes within a person's meaning-making system. As part of their recovery, people involved in this study reported radically changing a number of core beliefs they held about themselves, other people and their experience of distress.

At the start of their recovery journeys, people described a strong belief that they were negatively different to everyone else. They had no sense of their personal value and were consumed by feelings of powerlessness, lack of self-belief and, for some, self-hatred. Recovery first involved a gradual realisation of their value and innate resourcefulness. Initially, this sense of value came through the experience of being overtly valued by others and a realisation that each member of the group shared the same essential human nature. This sense of personal value was then developed through actively reaching out to others and by successfully learning how to tackle life problems.

People's perspectives on their power to bring about personal change or control their feelings also transformed. Prior to coming to GROW, people were entrapped by feelings generated by unresolved trauma that led to a deep sense of powerlessness. Life had become dangerous and the future no longer held any promise. Nothing they did seemed to make any difference. When they heard and saw the recovery testimonies of other people who had successfully escaped from similar places of terror, these beliefs were dramatically challenged. People soon began to realize that they had many resources for living and that they had the power to change their way of thinking and acting. Witnessing other people's recovery and experiencing the successful development of their own resources for living led to a genuine transformation in the way people dealt with life. Parts of the GROW program, such as 'I will go by what I know not by how I feel, and I will strive to improve my knowledge and understanding' (GROW 2001:10) or 'I can compel my muscles to act rightly in spite of my feelings' (GROW 2001:10), encouraged the development of reason which began to replace feelings and imagination that had for so long provided the basis for thinking. In this way, over time, people began to create radically new beliefs, such as 'I am more durable than vulnerable' (GROW 2001:32) rather than 'I am powerless'; 'the best in love, life and happiness is ahead of me' (GROW 2001:37) rather than 'there is no future for me'. Through trying out different life strategies and learning from these experiences, people gradually moved from a position of terrifying nihilism to a belief in the value of living a meaningful life and learned to see attractive possibilities for the future.

Having been let down by other people prior to GROW, many people had come to the belief that others were not to be trusted. These ideas affected their behaviour, feeding an intense desire to seek isolation in the belief that avoiding others would relieve their suffering. Experiencing inclusion in a compassionate community and being demonstrably valued by friendly others instilled a belief that [some] others could indeed be trusted. Instead of seeking the 'good' of isolation, as a possible means of escape from terror, participants increasingly realised the value of involvement with friendly and compassionate others and of learning to absorb tensions rather than seeking to avoid them. Instead of feeling powerless to deal with problems which fed the sense that 'they were no good', participants were empowered to tackle difficult situations and in this way began to realise their own power and worth, which was re-enforced by further actions involving befriending others, assuming leadership, working, volunteering and joining recreational groups.

Throughout the recovery process, participants began to change their beliefs about the nature and causes of 'mental illness' and recovery. People began to understand recovery as an educational process effected through reciprocal relationships with compassionate others rather than as a balancing of biochemistry which was dependent on the expertise of remote professionals. They reported realising that they, not the doctor, were primarily responsible for their own recovery and changed their understanding of medication from 'cure' to being a temporarily helpful form of external control, which could be replaced, over time, with other forms of self-care techniques, including relaxation, nutrition, exercise and healing friendships. They also began to re-frame their experience, viewing their experiential knowledge as a means of developing personal wisdom and character which could be used as a powerful source of help and support to others.

Engaging with the spiritual dimension of self

While spirituality was recognised by the participants as important to recovery and is regarded by some as the 'fourth dimension' of mental health care (Powell 2002, Cook 2011), it is seldom acknowledged within formal mental health services. Indeed, until recently, it was actively discouraged for fear that it might 'exacerbate symptoms such as religiously based content of hallucinations and delusions' (Starnino and Canda 2014:275). Powell (2002:1) suggests that the medical view of the human as essentially [nothing more than] a 'marvellous machine' controlled by a bio-chemically mediated mind leaves no room for concepts, such as the metaphysical soul, or indeed for the idea that people take unique meaning from their experiences. The findings of this study make it hard to ignore the idea that the person is essentially a spiritual being, one that lives within a series of bio/psycho and social bodies.

Chidarikire (2012:298) describes spirituality as 'the central way of life which guides people's conduct and is the essence of an individual's existence that integrates and transcends the physical, emotional, intellectual, volitional and social dimension'. Within Grow, spirituality is thought of in two ways: horizontal spirituality and vertical spirituality (GROW 2001:69). Horizontal spirituality can be defined as a source of human sustenance that comes through other people. It perhaps stems from a belief in the radical equality and value of every person and represents a form of care that brings life to each individual. People's narratives suggest that the human spirit was nourished by entering into the social womb of a mutual-support group. Through encountering compassionate and supportive others who warmly accepted and understood their wounded brokenness, seeds of hope, courage, endurance, warmth, understanding and goodness were planted deep within the hearts of each person. People also referred to a number of other things that they found spiritually sustaining and which they chose to develop in their own lives. Singing, dancing, studying, walking, appreciating nature, meditating, mindfulness, breathing techniques and doing good works were all quoted as valuable resources that helped fortify their spirit. Conversely, people described being stripped and drained of these same spiritual nutrients through the abuse and neglect of others to an extent that, prior to attending GROW, they lacked a belief in their own value, in the safety of the world and there being any point in living.

People's stories also revealed the importance of vertical spirituality. At the widest level, vertical spirituality addresses the whole question of belief in a higher being or power. Some participants openly professed a belief in God, a belief that helped them find meaning within all that had happened to them. Many people viewed God as some benign and eminent being who was concerned for them and who would providentially intervene in their lives. While others did not believe in a God, they all professed to believe in the healing power of 'goodness'. Goodness, in this context, meant believing in the power of consistently striving to be good, either by choosing to overcome obstacles in one's own life or by becoming involved in the 'good ordinary process' of helping others.

Concluding comments

This chapter has discussed eight recovery processes identified by people involved in this study which testify to the value of peer support in the lives of those experiencing and recovering from mental distress or 'mental illness'. Experiencing empathic and compassionate witness, becoming hopeful and believing in possibility, reconnecting with self and others, participating in positive and helpful risk taking, re-authoring a more positive identity, being the helper as well as the helped, transforming understanding of self and distress and engaging with the spiritual dimension of self are eight different processes which collectively released each person from a terrifying prison of isolation and slowly helped them become re-enchanted with their lives. In the same way that the microscope can be used to explore and understand pathological and healing processes involved in recovery from physical illness, this chapter acts as a lens through which processes of healing from mental distress can be understood, thus adding to the development of a non-medical and a more person-centred theory of recovery from a mutual-support perspective.

References

Amering, M. & Schmolke, M. 2009. *Recovery in mental health: Reshaping scientific and clinical responsibilities*, Oxford, Wiley Blackwell.

Bakhtin, M. 1981. *The dialogical imagination*, Austin, University of Texas Press.

Browne, I. 2008. *Music and madness*, Cork, Cork University Press.

Bruner, J. 2002. *Making stories: Law, literature, life*, Cambridge, MA, London, Harvard University Press.

Cain, C. 1991. Personal stories: Identity acquisition and self-understanding in Alcoholics Anonymous. *Ethos*, 19, 210–253.

Chamberlin, J. 1978. *On our own: Patient-controlled alternatives to the mental health system*, New York, McGraw-Hill.

Charon, R. 2006. *Narrative medicine: Honoring the stories of illness*, Oxford, Oxford University Press.

Chidarikire, S. 2012. Spirituality: The neglected dimension of holistic mental health care. *Advances in Mental Health*, 10, 298–302.

Clancy, L., Happell, B. & Moxham, L. 2014. The language of risk: Common understanding or diverse perspectives? *Issues in Mental Health Nursing*, 35, 551–557.

Coleman, R. 2004. *Recovery: An alien concept*, Fife, IL, P&P Press.

Cook, C. H. H. 2011. *Theology, transcendence and mental health*. Mental Health Practical Theology and Spirituality Conference. June 10, Dublin. All Hallows College.

Corrigan, P. W., Slopen, N., Gracia, G., Phelan, S., Keogh, C. B. & Keck, L. 2005. Some recovery processes in mutual-help groups for persons with mental illness. II: Qualitative analysis of participant interviews. *Community Mental Health Journal*, 41, 721–735.

Davidson, L., O'Connell, M. J., Tondora, J., Steaheli, M. & Evans, A. C. 2007. Recovery in serious mental illness: Paradigm shift or shiboleth? *Professional Psychology: Research and Practice*, 36, 480–487.

Deegan, P. 1995. Coping with recovery as a journey of the heart. *Psychiatric Rehabilitation Journal*, 19, 91–97.

Elliott, J. 2005. *Using narrative in social research: Qualitative and quantitative approaches*, Los Angeles, Sage.

Finn, L. D., Bishop, B. J. & Sparrow, N. 2009. Capturing dynamic processes of change in GROW mutual help groups for mental health. *American Journal of Community Psychology*, 44, 302–315.

Fisher, D. 2005. Empowerment model of recovery from severe mental illness: An expert interview with Daniel B. Fisher, MD, PhD. *Medscape Psychiatry & Mental Health*. Available at http://power2u.org/articles/recovery/expert_interview.html.

Frank, A. 1995. *The wounded storyteller: Body, illness, and ethics*, Chicago, University of Chicago Press.

Frank, A. W. 2002. *At the will of the body: Reflections on illness*, New York, Houghton Mifflin.

GROW 2001. *Program of growth to maturity*, Sydney, GROW Publications.

Higgins, A., Doyle, L., Downes, C., Morrissey, J., Costello, P., Brennan, M. & Nash, M. 2015. There is more to risk and safety planning than dramatic risks: Mental health nurses' risk assessment and safety-management practice. *International Journal of Mental Health Nursing*, 25(2), 159–170, doi: 10.1111/inm.12180.

Kartalova-O'Doherty, Y., Stevenson, C. & Higgins, A. 2012. Reconnecting with life: A grounded theory study of mental health recovery in Ireland. *Journal of Mental Health*, 21, 135–143.

Kennedy, M. 1995. *Becoming a GROWER: Worldview transformation in committed members of a mental health mutual help group*. Unpublished doctoral dissertation, Department of Educational Psychology, University of Illinois, DAI.

Kloos, B. 1999. *Cultivating identity: Meaning making in the context of residential treatment settings for persons with histories of psychological disorders*. Unpublished doctoral dissertation, University of Illinois at Urbana, Champaign IL.

Kuhn, T. S. 1962. *The structure of scientific revolutions*, Chicago, University of Chicago Press.

Lanius, R., Vermetten, E. & Pain, C. (eds.) 2010. *The impact of early life trauma on health and disease*, Cambridge, Cambridge University Press.

Leamy, M., Bird, V., Le Boutillier, C., Williams, J. & Slade, M. 2011. Conceptual framework for personal recovery in mental health: Systematic review and narrative synthesis. *The British Journal of Psychiatry*, 199, 445–452.

Loat, M. 2011. *Mutual support and mental health: A route to recovery*, London, Jessica Kingsley Publishers.

Maddock, S. & Hallam, S. 2010. *Recovery begins with hope*, London UK, National School of Government (Sunningdale Institute) & the Department for Business Innovation and Skills.

Morgan, J. F. 2007. *Giving up the culture of blame' risk assessment and risk management in psychiatric practice: Briefing document for Royal College of Psychiatrists*, London, Royal College of Psychiatrists.

Powell, A. 2002. *Mental health and spirituality*. Available at http://www.rcpsych.ac.uk/workinpsychiatry/specialinterestgroups/spirituality/publicationsarchive.aspx Accessed 30th November 2015.

Rappaport, J. 2000. Community narratives: Tales of terror and joy. *American Journal of Community Psychiatry*, 28, 1–24.

Riessman, F. 1965. The 'helper' therapy principle. *Social Work*, 10, 27–32.

Rogers, E. B. & Stanford, M. S. 2015. A church-based peer-led group intervention for mental illness. *Mental Health, Religion & Culture*, 18, 470–481.

Rose, N. 1998. Living dangerously: Risk-thinking and risk management in mental health care. *Mental Health Care*, 1, 263–266.

Rowan, J. & Jacobs, M. 2002. *The therapist's use of self*, Buckingham, Philadelphia, Open University Press.

Slade, M. 2009. *Personal recovery and mental illness: A guide for mental health professionals*, Cambridge, Cambridge University Press.

Starnino, V. R. & Canda, E. R. 2014. The spiritual developmental process for people in recovery from severe mental illness. *Journal of Religion & Spirituality in Social Work: Social Thought*, 33, 274–299.

Stuart, G. W. 2010. Mind to care and a future of hope. *Journal of the American Psychiatric Nurses Association*, 16, 360–365.

Thornicroft, G. 2006. *Discrimination against people with mental illness*, Oxford, Oxford University Press.

Wehmeyer, M. L. 1998. Self-determination and individuals with significant disabilities: Examining meanings and misinterpretations. *Research and Practice for Persons with Severe Disabilities*, 23, 5–16.

14 An exploration of recovery through graphic illustrations

The previous chapter explored eight processes that emerged from people's accounts of prolonged involvement in peer support. These processes nurtured and fuelled people's recovery, enabling each person's unique path to unfold naturally within the context of their emerging capabilities. This chapter presents a definition of recovery and explores three graphic illustrations that have been developed as a result of our listening to and engaging with the stories we heard.

Definition of recovery

From the exploration of people's stories, the following definition of recovery has been created:

> Recovery is a dynamic and ongoing educative process of personal transformation, effected through reciprocal relationships with compassionate but honest others. It involves self-activation, the taking of personal responsibility and the development of personal resources and support systems, which enable people to flourish and have a zest for living, even when life becomes challenging.

The nature of the person

The 'Nature of the Person' (Figure 14.1) seeks to depict the human being as a unique spirit embedded in a number of personal and social storytelling bodies, and to illustrate the relationship between the different processes involved in people's journey into severe emotional distress, and, subsequently, their journey towards recovery.

The person is viewed as a unique human spirit dwelling within a series of storytelling bodies. These storytelling bodies are in constant open dialogue with each other and exert influence on the person's decision-making processes and life direction. The first storytelling body is the 'personal' body of each unique individual, a body which internally generates physical, emotional and cognitive stories, which cyclically influence each other and give rise to a behavioural story of action. The person is also embedded within a social storytelling body, which includes family, friends and community. This storytelling body also interacts with and reciprocally influences stories generated within the personal storytelling body.

In addition, the person is located within wider local, national and international cultures and contexts, which also act as social storytelling bodies. Each culture, with its own unique set of rules, norms and values, not only impacts and influences the meaning the person attaches to their experience, but it shapes their actions and interactions. In other words, whilst the person may shape the culture and context of the world they live in, they are also shaped by it.

As a unique human being or 'unknowable spirit', both the personal and social storytelling bodies are also embedded within a cosmic creation, or what McFague (1993) calls the 'body of God' and which we have termed 'life's mystery'. In McFague's (1993:vii) view, the 'world is our meeting place with God, as the body of God it is wondrously, awesomely, divinely mysterious. God is not only transcendent but is immanently concerned with, and involved in, every single part of creation'. Irrespective of how the wider cosmos is conceptualised or named, it also attracts stories that become part of the person's story, such as stories that give meaning to suffering or lead to a belief in providence or divine intervention or other stories that may be used to explain or account for 'mystery'.

In the context of mental health, the diagram illustrates the complementary processes of emotional decline and emotional growth, processes that are constantly at work within each living person. It suggests that the journey towards severe emotional distress or 'mental illness' begins within the physical storytelling body of the individual, in response to negative or traumatic experiences, which act as an unexpected turning point or 'peripeteia' in the person's life (Bruner 2002). The immediate impact of these experiences is a dramatic non-verbal sensation or somatic story felt deep within the physical body of the person.

This somatic or physical story gives birth to many destructive emotions (terror, rage, resentment) and thoughts (mistrust of self and others), all of which undermine the person's ability to think rationally and ultimately disrupts their sense of control, flow and understanding of life. The person begins to doubt themselves and others, and start to develop patterns of 'catastrophic thinking' (Seligman 2007), ways of thinking which GROW (2001) suggests are unduly influenced by reactive feelings and imagination rather than considered reason and choice. These feelings and thoughts impact the person's behaviour causing, in many cases, the person to seek social isolation, a state which attracts other destructive cognitive and emotional stories and which excludes the person from the positive emotions and interactions necessary for healthy life and living. Consequently, the person's story becomes 'populated' with overwhelmingly negative feelings of despair, terror and powerlessness, which are cognitively translated or appropriated into a story of alienation and 'otherness'.

When the person seeks help for their distress within traditional mental health services, other cultural and professional stories associated with a medical diagnosis of 'mental illness' are added, which in many situations exacerbate a sense of despair, negative difference and otherness. As Bakhtin (1981:293) suggests, 'language is not a neutral medium that passes freely and easily into private property

The nature of a person: a human spirit dwelling within a series of personal and social storytelling bodies, which in turn exist within the context of life's mystery/the body of God. All are in constant open dialogue with each other and exert influence on the person's life direction.

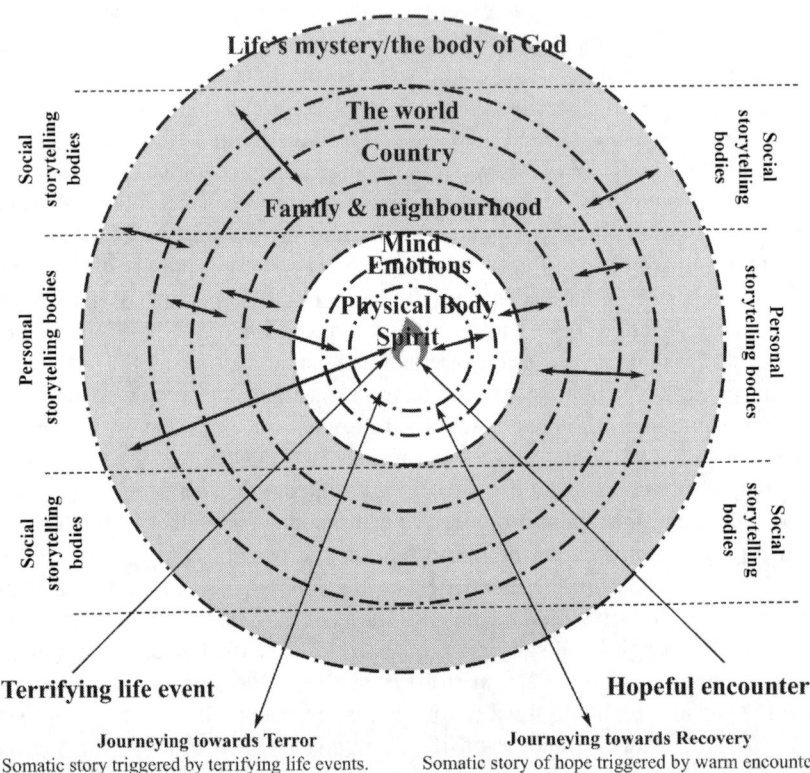

Terrifying life event   **Hopeful encounter**

Journeying towards Terror

Somatic story triggered by terrifying life events.
Absence of a caring or listening other.
Person's thoughts become protective, leading them towards withdrawal and isolation.
Isolation leads to thinking by feelings and imagination.
Emergence of levels of distress and chaos that lead to a diagnosis of "mental illness".
Diagnosis leads to cultural story of stigma, negative identity, and increased dependency on mental health professionals.

DESPAIR, SADNESS, FEAR, DARKNESS

Journeying towards Recovery

Somatic story of hope triggered by warm encounter with caring others.
Ongoing availability of empathic witness.
Thoughts become hopeful and awaken to possibilities leading towards reciprocal involvement.
Involvement leads to trust, open dialogue and shared responsibility for community.
Emergence of personal strength and growth.
Full participation in social roles and relationships.
Personal fulfillment and a desire to help others.
Person begins to flourish and develop a zest for life.

HOPE, JOY, MEANING, LIGHT

Figure 14.1 The nature of the person

of the speaker's intentions; it is populated – overpopulated-with the intentions of others'. In the case of emotional distress, the language of diagnosis is populated with feelings of shame and stigma. In this way, a story, which begins with an experience of distress and which includes being labelled as 'mentally ill' is 'spoken' at many levels, and over time plunges the person into 'chaos' or 'adventure time' (Bakhtin 1981).

The process of recovery through peer support is very similar to the one leading into profound distress and involves the same relationships between a life-changing somatic story and subsequent feelings, thoughts and actions; however, the direction is now working to reverse social withdrawal and distressing isolation. This time, the turning point or 'peripeteia' is a hopeful rather than a traumatic encounter, which enables the person to begin appropriating a different type of story. A warm and emotional welcome from caring and empathic others is first felt deep within the physical body and translated or appropriated into a positive somatic story of hope. The resultant feelings of hope begin to open up a world of new and attractive possibility and begin to effect the person's thinking, so that they can consider alternatives to isolation, even if they are, as Mags suggests, not 'capable of thinking that far ahead'. As the person is drawn into reciprocal involvement where they are befriended, unconditionally accepted and tangibly valued by a compassionate group, stories of hope, joy, belonging and personal value are attracted. Over time, these emotional stories are translated into thoughts that are increasingly 'populated' by the positive language of value, ability, power and belonging. Bakhtin (1981:345) describes these experiences as 'internally persuasive discourses', stories told inside the person at the emotional and cognitive levels but fuelled and endorsed by the behaviour or language of others. As the person leaves their cocoon of terror, discovers their own potential for leadership, and learns how to manage fears and do the 'good ordinary' thing, they begin to re-author or appropriate a different story of identity.

With each new achievement the person comes to a stage in their recovery where they develop an internally generated resilience. Here reliance on others is replaced by an enchanting sense of their own resourcefulness and, having served an 'apprenticeship' in living within a mutual peer-support group, the person is not only ready, but desires to assume a variety of roles with social niches in the community, which in turn attract other positive stories of identity.

Understanding the human being within the context of time

The diagram 'understanding the human person within the context of time' (Figure 14.2) offers the metaphor of the person as an ever-changing biological, psychological, social and spiritual being, with the ability to author and re-author his or her identity and life story. In this diagram, each person is once again depicted as a spirit living within a series of personal and social storytelling bodies, all of which exist within life's mystery. All these contexts themselves exist within a fourth dimension of time.

Words Made Flesh

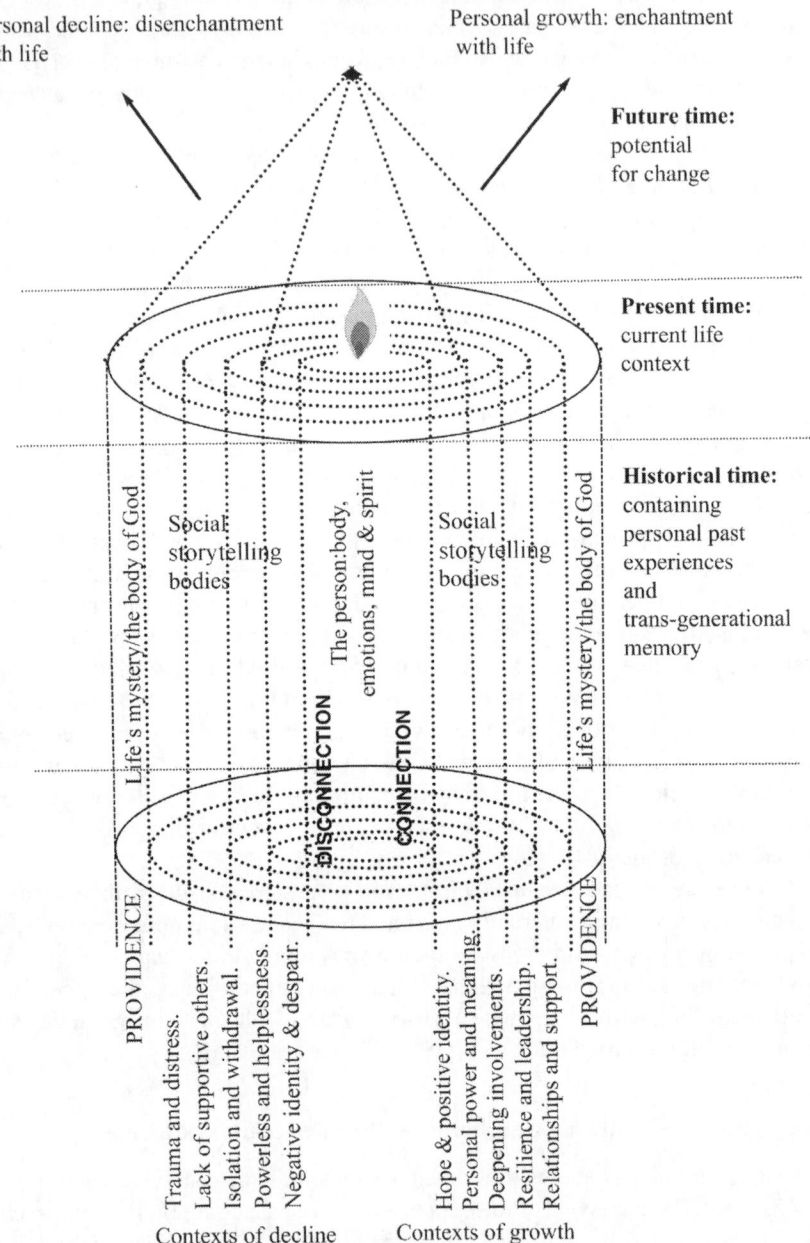

Figure 14.2 Understanding the human person within the context of time

Source: Adapted from Hoffman 1983:11

Time is depicted on a continuum ranging from a historical past to the present and into the future. Historical time stretches back through the person's life and beyond into eternity. Thus, historical time not only refers to the person's unique past experience but incorporates trans-generational memories and the whole story of an emergent humankind. Many theorists have suggested that each person has inherited a collective memory through the lived experiences of others. For Jung (1965) this is a 'collective unconsciousness', for Tolle (2005) it is an 'unconscious pain memory' and for Seligman (2007) a 'collective awareness of danger'. In this way, the past contains significant life events, but it also includes unique sets of values and interpretations specific to each individual's family, community, religion and culture.

Present time is about the current context of the person's life. It involves a person's current stage of growth or decline and includes their current life perspective, understandings, meanings, traumas, regrets and desires. It is also about their current sense of identity, power and control, the presence or absence of supportive and empowering relationships and the presence of immediate goals. The present is always 'pregnant' with potential and opportunity and can be the starting point for personal growth and recovery.

Time also extends beyond the present into future time. Future time is inhabited by dreams and aspirations and represents an opportunity to grow and develop, change, re-author and personally flourish. The diagram, shaped like an existential pencil, suggests that, irrespective of the past, each person has the potential to author and re-author their identity and life direction into the future.

The base of the diagram represents two opposing sets of contexts which conspire to influence a person's life direction, one towards personal growth and connection and the other towards personal decline and disconnection. The context for growth includes a positive sense of identity, a personal sense of hope and power and an ability to deal with life's inevitable stresses and strains. It also includes meaningful relationships with others and a sense of meaning and purpose in life. In the context of mental health and recovery, this context can be nurtured by the eight processes identified in the previous chapter, namely: experiencing empathic and compassionate witness, becoming hopeful and believing in possibility, reconnecting with self and others, participating in positive and helpful risk taking, re-authoring a more positive identity, being the helper as well as the helped, transforming understanding of self and distress and engaging with the spiritual dimension of self.

In contrast, the context for decline is rooted in personal feelings of despair, a lack of personal value and meaning, and a withdrawal from relationships with others and from life. People are devoid of the nurturing process required for healthy, connected living.

Irrespective of whether a person is moving along the pathway of growth and connection or decline and disconnection, their journey is still undertaken within the context of the mystery of life.

In the context of recovery, the diagram, which is inspired by Hoffman's (1983) Time Cable, can be used to initiate dialogue with the person, tracing the onset and impact of people's distress within the various contexts of their body, mind and relationships. It thus has the potential to facilitate compassionate discussion around a person's past experiences of life, their current stage of growth or decline, and their wishes, dreams or immediate recovery/life goals for the future, including what would assist in the construction of appropriate and positive pathways into the future.

Making a recovery map

The recovery map (Figure 14.3) places each person at the heart of a resourcefull local community which contains a multitude of potential social networks and resources for living. These diverse resources for living, which the persons themselves may be unaware of, or may be overlooked by mental health professionals, have the potential to support unique recovery pathways tailored to the emerging needs and desires of each person.

In this diagram, the person is portrayed as a universal warrior. The image of a warrior is not used to represent a person at war with the world or one who is destructive, dangerous or revengeful but to portray the potential of each person to show great vigour, courage and strength of spirit in overcoming life challenges and traumas and grow into the person they wish to become. For many, recovery will call people to personal heroism in overcoming fears and wounds from the past.

Each person or warrior carries with them a 'sword of truth', a descriptive model of the world which shapes their interactions with the world and which in turn evokes particular responses from that world. The sword of truth can be understood as a person's '*weltanschauung*', a term coined by philosopher Wilhelm von Humboldt (1767–1835) and defined by Sire (2009:15) as:

> a commitment, a fundamental orientation of the heart, that can be expressed as a story or in a set of presuppositions (assumptions which may be true, partially true, or entirely false), which we hold (consciously or subconsciously, consistently or inconsistently) about the basic construction of reality, and that provides the foundation on which we live and move and have our being.

Each warrior also carries a 'shield of friendship' representing their unique support network, people who will support and help the person overcome life's challenges and build resilience. This shield or friendly social body may be absent in the person's life, and it is this shield of friendly others that needs to be identified and developed in order to support the person in their recovery journey.

Thus, the recovery map (Figure 14.3) identifies possible pathways to any number of potential sources of help found in the person's local community. In a circular manner, it begins with family, friends and neighbours, and moves outwards to locally based peer-support groups. It includes short term courses and interventions that may be run by professionals, peers or a combination of both. It directs people to a whole range of other resources that may support their unique path in the context of their dreams and wishes, such as education, art, music, sport and

MAKING A RECOVERY MAP
using local resources

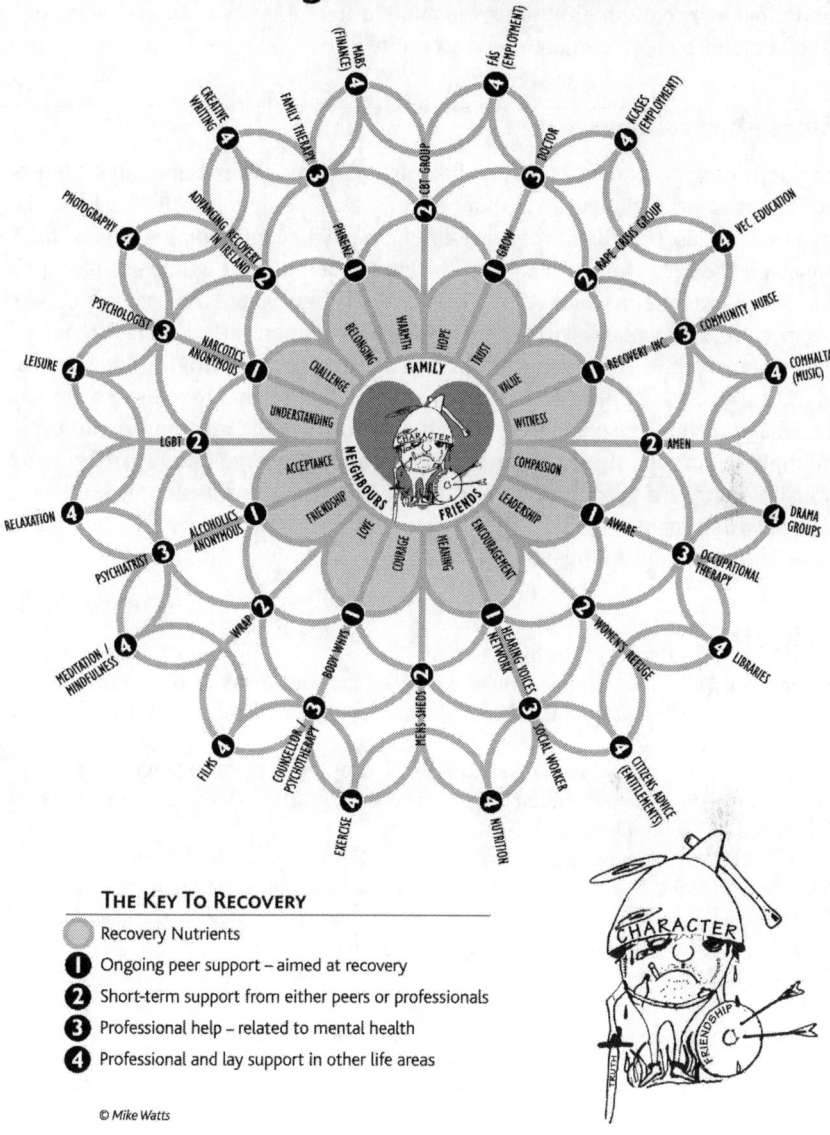

THE KEY TO RECOVERY

- Recovery Nutrients
- ❶ Ongoing peer support – aimed at recovery
- ❷ Short-term support from either peers or professionals
- ❸ Professional help – related to mental health
- ❹ Professional and lay support in other life areas

© Mike Watts

Figure 14.3 The recovery map

technology. The map also highlights a range of professional forms of support; however, professional support should always be based on the GROW maxim 'the expert should be on tap not on top' (GROW 2001:52). The recovery map, which can be adapted for each person's local context, may act as a point of discussion or guide for the person, highlighting the many different types of support and social involvements available in their local community.

Concluding comments

The definition of recovery and the diagrams that arose from our analysis of people's stories are included for a number of reasons. Pragmatically, we hope they may become useful aids to recovery-oriented practice, providing a way of thinking about the nature of recovery and the human being in the context of past, present and future time. As such, they may invite dialogue about the person's context, perspective, dreams and wishes. They may also support reflection on the impact, over time, of significant events in a person's life and subsequent life choices, leading to a speculative dialogue on the type of help that might prove most beneficial. The diagrams may also enable a reflective analysis of the relationship among the multiple factors that lead to mental distress and recovery and may offer a more holistic theory building base rather than some of the linear monologues which currently dominate and shape discussion on causes and treatment of 'mental illness' within the mental health services.

References

Bakhtin, M. 1981. *The dialogical imagination*, Austin, University of Texas Press.
Bruner, J. 2002. *Making stories: Law, literature, life*, Cambridge, MA, London, Harvard University Press.
GROW 2001. *Program of growth to maturity*, Sydney, GROW Publications.
Hoffman, L. 1983. A co-evolutionary framework for systemic family therapy. *Australian Journal of Family Therapy*, 4, 9–21.
Jung, C. G. 1965. *Memories, dreams, reflections*, New York, Random House.
McFague, S. 1993. *The body of god: An ecological theology*, Minneapolis, Fortress Press.
Seligman, M. E. P. 2007. *What you can change. . . . and what you can't: The complete guide to successful self-improvement*, New York, Vintage.
Sire, J. W. 2009. *The universe next door: A basic world view catalog*, Downers Grove, IL, Intervaristy Christian Fellowship.
Tolle, E. 2005. *A new earth create a better life*, London, Penguin.

15 Journey's end and new beginnings

The last chapter of this book brings to an end what has been a journey of discovery for us. It is a journey which has spanned a number of years and has been one of cooperative reflection and shared authorship. At times, it has been a difficult and challenging journey and, at other times, life enriching and exhilarating. Challenging because of the sheer responsibility of putting into words people's painful yet resilient stories; difficult because of the limitation of the written word, our own paucity of vision and expression and the immensity of concepts, such as the human being, time, providence, wellness and recovery. Life enriching because of our encounters with people who demonstrated such strength of spirit and life-giving generosity. Exhilarating as we uncovered ideas, such as the notion of 're-enchantment with life', and 'somatic stories' or became conscious that voices from philosophy, poetry and theology, as well as the human sciences, could illuminate what we were trying to understand and articulate. Writing the final chapter has also been a struggle, as the story is not finished.

Our struggle is no different to the struggle that has gone on since the beginnings of our common human history. Indeed, the mental health field has always been 'a space of contestation, struggle and resistance' (McDaid and Higgins 2014:270). Depending on epistemological and ontological perspectives, people have debated both the cause and treatment of mental distress and 'mental illness', producing numerous theories, academic papers, books and reflections, all laying claim to some form of unique wisdom and insight. As discussed at the beginning of this book, common to many of the explanatory frameworks and prescriptive solutions is the idea that mental distress or 'mental illness' is some form of 'objective phenomenon' caused by a personal pathology located within the individual. As such, mental distress is seen as a pathology which exists devoid of context, relevance and meaning and which requires 'expert' interventions from a 'knowing', paid other, who has undergone a period of professional education and training in the latest theory or intervention. As a direct consequence, the majority of contemporary mental health services around the world are structured in a manner that not only privileges the voice and stories of those in positions of power and authority but effectively gives the educated 'other' power over the people who come or are brought to the service seeking help. In doing so, the stories of the people who should be at the heart of the service become submerged within a plethora of professional theories and perspectives. Consequently, other potential stories of meaning and recovery arising from outside these socially and legally sanctioned structures get silenced, marginalised or ignored or simply remain unheard within mainstream mental health service provision.

We are very aware that it is always easy to critique the past or deconstruct ideologies that do not sit with one's own perspective. It is much more difficult, however, to develop or create an alternative narrative to the one traditionally perpetuated within mainstream mental health and psychiatry. Whilst this book is an attempt to offset some of the professional hegemony that surrounds discussion on mental health and potential for recovery, we are not endeavouring to discount all professionally driven mental health services or insights gained from social sciences, psychiatry, nursing or other disciplines. Neither are we trying to position peer support in opposition to psychiatry and professional help, nor are we trying to suggest that peer support will work for everyone.

Arising from an interpretive epistemology, using a narrative methodology, a less researcher-centric way of doing research, this book is about enabling some of the silent and untold stories to breathe aloud and be heard. Unlike many professionally driven discourses on mental distress, where people's experience is framed from the outset with the context and language of illness, diagnosis, symptoms and disability, this book is an attempt to tell a different type of story. Based on an analysis of the stories of our 26 co-authors as they recovered from experiences of what were labelled 'mental illnesses' through their involvement in GROW, the primary focus is on the very rich and moving accounts of each person's journey to 're-enchantment with life'. The story told through the words of the people interviewed focuses on their perspectives and the meaning they attach to their experiences as they moved from a place of disconnection, despair and isolation to a place of personal empowerment and liberation through peer support. Whilst being a story of vulnerability, trauma, hurt and pain, it is also a story of hope, meaning, strength, empathy, respect, spirituality and above all, a story of healing through reciprocal relationships and shared responsibility. Importantly, it is also a story of how mental distress can be constructed as part of the human experience and condition as opposed to viewing this distress as an illness with symptoms. It is a story of how distress can be overcome when people are in an environment where the emphasis is on listening, empathic witness and personal recognition as opposed to naming, labelling and categorising. Hopefully, in a time when protocols, algorithms and prescriptive approaches are increasingly gaining momentum within psychiatry, it is a story that highlights the importance of providing people with an environment that nurtures, supports, challenges and scaffolds their recovery journeys in a way that enables each person's unique path to unfold naturally within the context of their emerging capabilities, plans and dreams for the future.

Frank (2004) argues that many people experience a gap between what they know and what they can articulate, which can be a source of powerlessness, as 'what cannot be said cannot be acted on' (Frank 2004:437). In addition to articulating people's stories of recovery, which hopefully will act as points of inspiration and hope and a validation of people's experiences, we hope that these stories of recovery within the GROW community also give other complex issues an articulated form. Each story clearly illustrates that mental health issues do not occur in a vacuum but within the context of a network of destructive relationships and a lack of support and as such, recovery and healing is described by us as a dynamic and ongoing, educative process of personal transformation, effected through reciprocal relationships with compassionate and honest others. It involves self-activation, the taking of personal responsibility, and the development of personal resources and support systems, which enables people to flourish and have a zest for living, even when life becomes challenging.

In other words, recovery can be experienced as an ongoing dance that takes place within each person's heart and soul and which spills out towards others. It is a dance that has the potential to reveal each person's inestimable worth and generate the spiritual nutrients of wisdom, courage and endurance that we all need as we collectively struggle with the immense joys and the terrifying realities of life. It is a dance that takes place at multiple levels, inside and outside each human being, and is nurtured by processes such as experiencing empathic and compassionate witness, becoming hopeful and believing in possibility, reconnecting with self and others, participating in positive and helpful risk taking, re-authoring a more positive identity, being the helper as well as the helped, transforming understanding of self and distress and engaging with the spiritual dimension of self.

By revealing some of the processes that enable the natural unfolding of people's recovery journey, the stories also shine a light on the fundamental differences between relationships that occur within traditional mental health services and those that occur in a peer- or mutual-support context. While peer-support organisations may differ in focus, they are all grounded in what Scott et al. (2011:188) calls 'the peer's liminal position', as peers are both inside and outside the experience of 'madness'. As demonstrated throughout the stories, peer support, unlike relationships within the psychiatric service, is underpinned by a non-hierarchical mode of being with people who all had similar struggles. People engaged with peer support do 'not exist in a subordinate position of power' relative to the other (Adame and Leitner 2008:149), and neither are they cast as the 'ill other'. Within peer support, by being both givers and receivers, people bear equal responsibility for the healing of one another. Similarly, the strength of peer support lies in the acknowledgment of everyone's vulnerability and brokenness, as well as the power that comes from revealing oneself to others. In the context of the emerging model of recovery-oriented services, this poses real challenges for the professions involved in mental health care. If practitioners are to develop an emotionally embodied way of being with the self and others which acknowledges the shared humanity of all, there is a need for a radical shift away from the current focus on hiding and protecting vulnerabilities, minimising or avoiding personal disclosure and having power over the other. All of us working in the arena of mental health need to develop a way of being and a 'generosity of spirit' (Frank 2004) that enables us to bear witness to pain and suffering and engage compassionately with people as equally valuable human beings. There is also a need for us to recognise the wisdom and expertise that each person carries about their own life and recovery, which if listened to can collectively improve our knowledge of human distress and recovery.

People's stories of recovery told within the pages of the book also challenge one of the edifices that currently underpins the whole of the psychiatric health system, namely, the use of diagnosis. The stories narrated not only highlight the often destructive nature of both the diagnosis and the manner of its delivery, but once again remind us that diagnosis, which may be helpful for some, like a double-edged sword has the power to discount meaning and context, shape identities and rob the person of hope and any sense of future. Once labelled, the person's story of trauma and the context of their lives get discounted, as they quickly become transformed into a passive, objective 'other' with a negative identity that is toxically rooted deep within our cultural mind. By framing the person's story and life contexts within the fixed meaning of diagnosis, the personal story gets submerged (Barker 2003), unheard and unwitnessed, and the opportunity to commence a real dialogue that might prompt a personal voyage of discovery and recovery is almost certainly lost.

The stories, as told by our 26 co-authors, also raise questions about the role of practitioners in a recovery-oriented mental health service. Their stories clearly demonstrate that participation in intelligently selected social niches provides people with opportunities to author alternative positive identities, eroding any sense of negative difference and fulfilling a deep need within people to have a meaningful place in life, in addition to exposing them to other attractive life possibilities. The challenge for the mental health services lies in creating cooperative pathways with people in recovery and the host of agencies outside mainstream mental health services that will enable meaningful engagement with society, in accordance with people's emerging needs and dreams.

While recognising that peer relationships are different to practitioner–service user relationships and can never be fully replicated within a professional context, the stories of recovery presented in this book do raise the question of why peer support is still on the margins or periphery of the mainstream mental health services. While the benefits of peer support are well recognised and valued by professionals within the fields of physical health, such as diabetes, asthma and cancer, peer-support interventions are not commonly part of a recovery plan for people experiencing mental distress. Today, the demand on mental health systems around the world far exceeds capacity, yet many mental health practitioners continue to operate in a professional-centric manner and fail to engage in a dialogue with peer-support services or provide information to people experiencing distress on how to access them. While peer support may not appeal to everyone, it represents a vast, untapped resource that can and should enrich the work of professionals and should therefore be viewed as adding to rather than competing with what they do. It is also a vast resource for people who may not wish to have their experience of distress framed within the traditional psychiatric model of 'mental illness' or those who may, for other reasons, wish to disengage from mainstream mental health services. Hence the need for mental health services and peer organisations to engage in mutually enriching conversations about how to work together. Whilst it is important for mental health services to work with peer support and support their development through the provision of funding and other resources, peer services need to be mindful of the risks of being co-opted or colonised by professional thinking and restrictions.

In conclusion, in setting forth our thinking and arguments, some people might say that this book is no different to what has gone before and is merely proffering and seeking to privilege another form of wisdom or dogma, this time derived from the lived experience of 26 people. They might argue that by the very act of writing the book we are already positively predisposed towards mutual help and support, a stance which not only influenced the questions we asked but subsequently shaped the manner in which coherence and order were brought to the stories told in previous chapters. Others might argue that the people involved were in no way representative of the 'average GROW person', and being seasoned members and having held numerous leadership positions, they were privileged elites themselves. Anyone with a cursory knowledge of research could also argue that the findings may be influenced by bias: those who benefited stayed in GROW and were happy to be interviewed, and those who did not left and we know nothing of their perspective. Others might point out that the GROW members who participated in the study had particular agendas and wished to portray the support in a very positive light, whilst others may highlight that the age profile is not representative, with an absence of young people's voices, or that the stories are subject to recall bias. If one wishes to view the book through a positivist lens and apply the cannons of research developed from that perspective, then all of these arguments are certainly valid. However, the story of recovery as narrated in the various chapters is located within a different research tradition, and as such we are not laying claims to generalisability or any of the other cannons that certain research traditions hold dear. For us, the fundamental questions around method and methodology are: Did we give an ethical hearing to people's stories? Did we do justice in our articulation to the deep wounds of people's distress and the complex nature of their journeys? And does the book have resonance for people who have, or are currently experiencing, mental distress?

Whilst we have no control over how people will read and interpret the text or indeed how they may use it in the future to argue a position, we hope that the book will act as a 'standpoint' to attract agreement and disagreement and in doing so not only contribute to the an ongoing exploration and debate around recovery and peer support but, more importantly, contribute to the development and enrichment of the services for people experiencing mental distress. We also hope that the book will give people, especially those working in the mental health service, both practitioners and policy makers, a framework for understanding the nature of peer support and the intricate process that nurtures people in their recovery. In doing so we hope that the book has revealed some of the often unquestioned and unspoken practices and interactions that occur within the mental health service and provided food for thought on how people can change their way of being with people in distress.

We also hope that the book holds relevance for everyone who is currently engaged in the many peer-support organisations that exist, providing a platform for conscious reflection about methodologies and the possibilities inherent in greater collaboration among peer support, professional help and society in general.

Finally, we hope that the book will be of practical use to people currently experiencing 'mental distress' and who have received a diagnosis of 'mental illness' and to those friends and family members who want to know how they can be of help. It would be nice if the stories contained within these chapters were to plant seeds of hope in the hearts of people currently wrestling with distress and trauma and were to help them start out on new journeys of recovery leading to 'a re-enchantment with life'. To conclude:

> We told our stories – That's all.
> We sat and listened to each other
> and heard the journeys of each soul.
> We heard love's longing
> and the lonely reachings-out
> for love and affirmation.
> We heard of dreams
> Shattered.
> And visions fled.
> Of hopes and laughter
> turned stale and dark.
> We felt the pain of
> isolation and
> the bitterness of death.
> But in each brave and
> lonely story
> God's gentle life
> broke through
> And we heard music
> in the darkness
> and smelt flowers
> in the void.
>
> Edwina Gateley
> (1999 with permission)

References

Adame, A. L. & Leitner, L. M. 2008. Breaking out of the mainstream: The evolution of peer support alternatives to the mental health system. *Ethical Human Psychology and Psychiatry*, 10, 146–162.

Barker, P. 2003. The Tidal Model: Psychiatric colonization, recovery and the paradigm shift in mental health care. *International Journal of Mental Health Nursing*, 12, 96–102.

Frank, A. W. 2004. After methods, the story: From incongruity to truth in qualitative research. *Qualitative Health Research*, 14, 430–440.

Gateley, E. 1999. *The sharing in psalms of a lay woman (new edition)*. Lanham, MD, The Rowman & Littlefield Publishing Group Inc.

McDaid, S. & Higgins, A. 2014. Into the future: Promoting mental health and democratising support for people with mental/emotional distress. *In*: Higgins, A. & McDaid, S. (eds.) *Mental health in Ireland: Policy, practice and law* (pp. 270–284), Dublin, Gill & Macmillan.

Scott, A., Doughty, C. & Kahi, H. 2011. 'Having those conversations': The politics of risk in peer support practice. *Health Sociology Review*, 20, 187–201.

Index